NUTI
F

MW00488657

Smart food choices
that can lower your score.

The key to
enhancing stamina,
improving concentration,
controlling temper.

by
Nina Anderson, Cherie Tripp & Dr. Howard Peiper
in cooperation with Neil Orenstein, Ph.D.

Foreword by
Patrick Bowers
Director of Golf,
Whistler Resort, British Columbia, Canada

Edited by Arlene Murdock, Heather and Stanley Rosenfeld

No part of this book may be reproduced in any form without
the written consent of the publisher

ISBN 1-884820-53-0
Library of congress Catalog Card Number 99-72917
Printed in the United States of America

Nutritional Leverage for Great Golf is not intended as medical advice. It is written solely for informational and educa-
tional purposes. Please consult a health professional should
the need for one be indicated.

Published by ATN Publishing
P.O. Box 36
East Canaan, CT 06024
(860) 824-5301

FOREWORD

As golfers, we know the sport's great advantage over many others is that it can be played and more importantly enjoyed, long into one's 80s, even with health complications. We have taught many individuals who have or had heart ailments or some form of cancer, who started playing golf as part of their recovery fitness program. One's golf game can continue to show improvement, which is gratefully reflected in a satisfying score.

Nutritional Leverage For Great Golf can help with that improvement. I found it to be an important guide, incorporating choices that are easy to follow, and ones that will positively contribute to better overall physical and mental performance on the course.

During the years that I have played, I have observed golfer's rituals and superstitions. I've seen anything and everything including "lucky" articles of clothing and talking to one's clubs, not to mention spiritual begging for par. I also have found that most players have conditioned eating and drinking patterns. I've witnessed radical performance changes, from distant hitting to putting. Players get increasingly frustrated when this happens, which only compounds the margin for error. It is now possible to consider that the root of some of these performance problems could be associated with what was eaten 20 minutes to 4 hours before taking to the course. It seems that even the pro-circuit tour players are becoming aware of the benefits of nutrition. In the Master's division, enlightenment probably resulted from health problems. There is Jack Nicklaus' hip replacement, cancer survivors like Palmer, and the long list of players with heart complications, etc., successfully pursuing tournament wins. They, like all of us, probably think about life-style changes to improve their health. Let's face it, if you feel well, you play well, and your score reflects that improvement.

For those looking to nutritionally support their ability to play a better golf game, this book may pinpoint the supportive foods now missing from their diets. For those interested in taking a more active role in enhancing their physical and mental performance, this book presents a common-sense approach that can easily be incorporated into anyone's lifestyle.

Nutritional Leverage for Great Golf also outlines some of the most prevalent ailments that we hear about from our players, such as back pain, and offers nutritional suggestions for healing and sickness prevention. The bonus travel chapter meets the challenge of destination golf resorts, focusing on information regarding jet lag, hot weather conditions in either deserts or the tropics, and altitude sickness and playing in mountain resorts.

Nutritional Leverage For Great Golf is a must-read for golfers of all skill levels, with key information for those who not only want to lower their score, but stay healthy as well.

-Patrick Bowers, Director of Golf, Whistler Resort, British Columbia, Canada

Acknowledgements.

In appreciation for their contribution to creating this book, we extend our gratitude to
Fred White, for his idea that sparked this book;
Dr. Uma Viswanathan, for her expertise;
Heather and Stanley Rosenfeld, for their professional editorial input;
Bob Stack, for his knowledge pertaining to the sport of golf;
Peter Lejeune, for his editorial skills; and
Nick Smith, for introducing us to the need for managing blood sugar during exercise.

INTRODUCTION

Golfers, like many athletes, have momentary breakdowns in concentration, and control of their physical body. A lower score versus too many bogeys, depends not only on athletic training, but also on the condition of one's physical body and state of mind. Many books guide one through physical conditioning exercises, the power of positive thinking, visualization, and other mind exercises specifically tailored to the golfer. It is critical to remember that weighing the merit of advice from the "pros" regarding different golf clubs and stroke control, is only part of the equation to improve, and more importantly, enjoy one's game.

Today, valuable nutritional information resulting from ever-increasing research, is available to improve one's health and sporting performance. *Nutritional Leverage for Great Golf* is based on studies that are well documented. Leading health advocates and organizations, like the American Heart Association (for example), herald much of the food choice information.

Nutritional Leverage for Great Golf focuses on nutrition and how it affects your body's performance. Some of this information may be familiar, while other recommendations may dispel long standing myths about diet. Also presented are new ways to use foods that can have a strong influence not only on your game, but your long-term health as well.

In addition to the recommendations in this book, we encourage you to maintain a fitness program. It is also advisable to follow an appropriate stretching regime, prior to each golf outing. We cover the nutrient portion of a diet, but always keep in mind that adding mind control, exercise, relaxation and laughter, make for a great personal improvement for the whole being.

-the authors

Table of Contents

SECTION 1. PERFORMANCE NUTRIENTS

SECTION 1. PERFORMANCE NUTRIENTS

Chapter 1. Water and electrolytes. The first step to improving concentration and muscle control.

It is scientific fact that you can live without food for quite some time, but not without water. Golfers *must* drink water while on the course. The fresh air, wind and sun rapidly dehydrate the body through perspiration and exhalation. Most clubs have well-documented stories of golfers who have suffered from acute dehydration. At the Canon Greater Hartford Open in 1999, it was reported that some of the players needed to have emergency medical treatment after playing in the extreme heat.

Know the symptoms of dehydration:
- memory lapse
- light-headedness
- breathing problems
- headaches

These are conditions that can ruin your golf game, not to mention compromising your overall health. The best preventive medicine is also the simplest—drink water! Without water, joints don't move, blood (contains 90% water) doesn't flow, and our body's organs don't work. Water makes up 85% of a baby's body, 60-67% of a full-grown man's body, 50-60% of a woman's body, and 75% of the human brain. In addition, water helps to regulate our body temperature, removes wastes, carries nutrients and oxygen to cells, and moistens our lungs, enabling us to breathe.

Without water, the brain doesn't think, and allow us to make judgments properly. This affects the golfer's swing, distance and direction. Water is also necessary to maintain strong muscles, which all golfers need to walk the 9-18 holes, or just to get in and out of the golf cart. Muscle tissue is comprised of approximately 75% water. Consistent swing control and overall hitting accuracy are dependent on muscles that have been hydrated.

Most physicians and nutritionists, along with golfers like *Don Tinder*, in his book *The Fitness for Golfers Handbook*, recommend drinking 8 glasses of water a day. Sugared drinks, coffee, alcohol and soda do not qualify. You must drink water. Coffee and colas are particularly risky, because the caffeine actually facilitates dehydration. If you absolutely have to have your coffee, follow it up with a chaser of 8 ounces of plain water. Alcohol also can dehydrate you, therefore we recommend on day of play, to reduce or restrict your intake of alcoholic beverages.

Dietitian consultant, Sally Girvan, explains that although alcohol is a traditional social aspect of golf, it can cause dehydration and affect concentration. (From the Pure Golf Academy website[1].)

Our beverage choice is bottled or filtered water with added electrolytes. We caution against tap water unless it has been filtered, as bacteria, chlorine (anti-bacterial), and chemicals have been detected in many city water supplies. Bottled water is safer, although you should check on the many report cards that have been made available to the public (see footnote)[2], which rates their quality.

Bottled waters, as previously stated, are not created equal. The Natural Resources Defense Council (NRDC) performed a test on bottled water producers to determine contaminants present in their product. Many companies exceeded the recommended levels for bacteria, arsenic and TTHMs (potentially cancer-causing chemicals created when organic matter reacts with chlorine). For purifying your water at home, there are numerous point-of-use filters available through supermarkets, hardware and plumbing supply stores, mail order and online

---

[1] www.golf.com.au/fitness/nutrition. Sally Girvan, consultant dietitian for the Australian Professional Golfers' Association.

[2] www.nrdc.org/nrdcpro/bw/appa.html Reports Bottled Water, Pure Drink or Hype? Select: Test Results: bottled water contaminants found. (202) 289-6868

catalogs. Travel filters are also available, so you can avoid the highly chlorinated water found in most hotels. Note that not all filters are equally efficient. Some devices remove sediment, others additionally remove chemicals and chlorine, while reverse-osmosis and distillation devices eliminate almost all contaminants including beneficial minerals. Most of our water, both tap, filtered and bottled, is mineral-deficient.

Our bodies depend on certain electrically charged minerals (electrolytes) to maintain the balance and flow of vital body fluids, transmit nerve impulses, and maintain healthy muscle function to operate the circulatory system. These electrolytes control the body's pH (acid/base) balance, and they facilitate transport of nutrients and waste products in and out of the cells. Most food produced today lacks these essential trace elements (missing from overworked farm soil), and failure to supplement one's mineral requirements can lead to the following symptoms:

•anemia •bone loss •blood-sugar problems •fatigue •gray hair •irregular heartbeat •low sperm count •muscle cramps •senility •wrinkles

Hospital physicians test for electrolyte levels as part of their diagnostic procedure. Hospital patients, many times, receive an electrolyte solution. This facilitates re-hydration and restoration of mineral balance. The nervous system is the communication system of the body. The brain and other sensors are the "computers". Unless this whole electro-chemical system is in balance, you cannot optimize your performance.

Exercise, and the inevitable sweat, evaporate electrolytes out of your body. To facilitate quick rehydration, electrolyte drinks were introduced to the sports marketplace years ago, primarily targeting professional football and baseball players. Sales of sports drinks with electrolytes added have soared tremendously with the help of high-profile celebrity endorsements from stars in the U.S. such as *Mia Hamm* and *Michael Jordan*.

Athletes know the importance of rehydration. If you don't replace electrolytes, your brain will not generate the proper electrical charge necessary to send accurate messages through the nervous system to your muscles, (for example, while you are swinging your club).

One mineral specifically tied to muscle coordination is potassium. This is an electrolyte that conducts electricity when dissolved in water. Deficiencies can arise from perspiration, and from replacing potassium-rich foods such as sunflower seeds, avocados, spinach and carrots, with foods most commonly eaten during hot weather such as carbonated beverages, ice cream, alcohol, fast foods and sugary snacks. Taking diuretics can also cause a deficiency. Low levels of potassium may affect the contraction process of the muscle, which may result in reduced control.

The optimum is to drink mineral water several times a day. If you keep hydrated by drinking mineralized water, wishing for a more precise game becomes more realistic, as your brain and muscles coordinate more efficiently.

Choosing a mineral product:

Mineral waters are easy to find wherever bottled water is sold. Brands such as Perrier, Vittel, S. Pellegrino, Dasani, Hildon, Gerolsteiner, Fiuggi, Crystal Geyser, Apollinaris and Calistoga, to name just a few, are labeled specifically as mineral water. These are selections you can either get from a soda vending machine or the beverage carts on many courses. Spring water does not necessarily contain minerals, therefore if you want to get adequate electrolytes, choose the brands that say mineral water.

If you are considering mineral supplements, you need to select ones in a form (molecular size) that permeate the cell membrane. These should contain all the necessary trace minerals (there are many other minerals that your body can't use). Mineralized cells are receptive, hard workers that provide your brain with maximum performance.

Colloidal minerals should be avoided, as they are the largest form and are considered less effective at permeating the cell membrane because they are too big. Chelated and ionic minerals are smaller than colloidal, and have a better chance of being absorbed. Chelation is the process of bonding a mineral to an amino acid in supplement form (not liquid). This bonding makes it easier to digest and assimilate for proper utilization in the body. Crystalloid is the name for the homeopathic form of ionic minerals, scaled very small to optimize permeating the cell membrane.

When choosing a supplement, it is very difficult to ascertain if the minerals are colloidal unless the label identifies them. If you purchase supplements at a pharmacy, you may ask the druggist to steer you to the preferred brands. Most health food stores carry brands that identify colloidal on the label. Supplements come in pill form, and in a liquid which can mix readily in your water bottle.

Quick reference notes:

➤Symptoms of dehydration are memory lapse, light-headedness, breathing problems, and headaches.

➤Lack of water short-circuits our brain

➤Water is necessary to maintain strong muscles.

➤Exercise, sweating, alcohol and caffeine dehydrate us.

➤Drink mineral water or purified water with added electrolytes to prevent dehydration when exercising.

➤Bottled water is not always healthy. Check out the website: *www. nrdc.org* or call (202)-289-6868 to find out which bottlers have contaminant-free water

➤Sports drinks with electrolytes are good.

➤Sports drinks with sugar added may give you a burst of energy followed by fatigue an hour or two later.

➤Symptoms associated with electrolyte (mineral) deficiencies are fatigue, anemia, bone loss, senility, muscle cramps, irregular heartbeat, low sperm count and impotence in men, blood-sugar problems, obesity, gray hair, wrinkles and lots more.

➤Electrolyte deficiencies arise from eating mineral-deficient food and water, dehydration and sweating.

➤The mineral potassium supports muscle coordination. Deficiencies stem from use of diuretics, from perspiration and from a diet of potassium-low foods, including carbonated beverages, ice cream, alcohol, fast foods and sugary snacks. Eat potassium-rich foods such as sunflower seeds, avocados, peanuts, raisins, spinach, potatoes, and carrots to name a few. Supplementation may also be necessary.

➤Mineral water (bottled) is a great choice to supplement your daily intake of purified water.

Chapter 2. Foods and performance.

Advice from the golf world, whether it is from magazines, books, videos, resident club or course pros, and golf school directors, centers on exercises, stroke training and mental techniques to improve our game. These are all important, but if the body is not nutritionally supported, it undermines all those hours of practice driving, chipping, putting, and mental conditioning.

Extreme-sports athletes are welded to strict nutrition regimens. On the surface, golf looks tame, but it too offers challenges, such as making that 16' putt on a wet rise, or seeking deliverance in a grove of trees positioned 2 feet apart, with 250 yards to the pin, and it is your 2nd shot for a par 4 hole. The golfer's body demands quality nutrients to carry out proper physical and mental control, similar to the "iron" men and women athletes. After all, it is a sport that demands concentration and performance levels to be sustained for two to four hours, depending on course traffic and the number of holes played.

The standard cliché, "you have to start a little at a time to change a life-time of habits", applies here as well. But, once you begin using these food recommendations, you will feel a positive change, both on and off the course. You may even want to recommend some tips to your golfing companions, especially those who like testing their carbon clubs on oak trees, or muttering expletives, often after every putt. In the following chapters, we will explain in detail, the benefits of the foods and supplements listed and how they can improve your golf life.

For those who have medical conditions and/or food allergies and are on restricted diets, or suspect they have a physical problem, please consult with your health practitioner.

The basic plan.

If you are like most of us, we have spent a lifetime eating certain foods because we were raised on traditional family meals. We also choose new foods based on print or television advertisements, cookbook recipes or a restaurant menu. Fast foods or microwave meals can be your answer to nutritious eating, or your diet may be strict organic vegetarian. The bottom line is, that everyone has different tastes, and each of our bodies react differently to foods and drink.

Alex McIntrye, Director of Golf at the Essex Golf & Country Club in LaSalle, Ontario, (Host Club of the 1998 Du Maurier Classic, one of the 4 major events on the LPGA tour), doesn't like to eat on the golf course. Alex feels it changes his sugar levels, so he plays hungry, only drinking fluids with electrolytes added. *Mel Sole*, Director of Instruction at the Phil Ritson, Mel Sole Golf School at Pawley's Plantation, in South Carolina prefers to snack on bananas, raisins, an energy bar, and an electrolyte drink. *Bob Wyatt, Jr.*, National coordinator Master Teaching Professional for the United States Golf Teachers Federation, also advises snacking on bananas and raisins. All of these teaching professionals advise a light pre-game meal, consisting only of fruit and grain products.

These personal choices are on the right track, but as you will come to understand in subsequent chapters, they are only adequate for specific conditions. The plan we outline below will get you started. We recommend sticking with it for two weeks and during that period, you will need to observe how you feel. If you notice a positive change, then you can transition to the TEE TIME menus described in Chapter 6.

Every golfer's body is different. Those who are religious about junk foods and candy bars may be resistant to changing their diet. But, if you want to lower your score, improve your concentration, have more stamina and feel generally better, this program is worth the two-week effort.

This diet was constructed in collaboration with Neil Orenstein, Ph.D., formerly affiliated with the Massachusetts General Hospital and Beth Israel Hospital (Harvard Medical School) in Boston. Neil maintains a private practice in Nutritional Biochemistry, working with people to reestablish their biochemical balance, in Lenox, MA. He may be reached at (413) 637-3466.

The Great Golf 2-week high-performance plan.

• Beverages:
> ►purified water (8 glasses per day)
> ►lemon juice in water (unsweetened lemonade)
> ►mineral water (minimum of 3 glasses per day)
> ►unsweetened vegetable juice (preferably those with low sodium or any freshly-juiced vegetable juice)

> *Avoid:*
> ►sugared drinks (no diet sugars, either)
> ►fruit drinks
> ►caffeine and alcohol, if possible.
> *If you are an avid coffee drinker, try to cut down, and follow each cup with a chaser of 8oz. water (avoids dehydration). If you must have alcohol, try to limit your daily consumption to 1 glass of beer or wine.*

22

- Foods:

  (examples only - partial list)
  - fish, chicken, turkey
  - yogurt (unsweetened)
  - cheese (without hydrogenated oil)
  - vegetables
  - potatoes, rice, pasta
  - beans (all legumes such as lentils or chick peas),
  - nuts
  - dark breads (whole grain, rye, pumpernickel, oat, spelt, rice)
  - unsweetened whole grain cereals (rice, oat meal, buckwheat, millet, corn grits, whole wheat)
  - fruit

  Avoid:
  - cereal with sugar added
  - foods with sugar as an ingredient
  - refined flour products (white bread)
  - fast foods
  - reduce intake of red meat (disrupts pH balance, contributing to potential mineral loss)
  - sugared desserts

• Snack foods:

Snack foods for sustained energy
► apples, grapes, plums, pears, cherries, citrus fruit
► peanuts
► granola (with oats and without sugar added)
► dark flour bread or muffins (without sugar added)
► unsweetened yogurt
► slow-release energy bar
► mineral water

Snack foods for quick energy.
► raisins, bananas, pineapple, watermelon
► rice cakes
► carrots (medium-release, can fit both categories)
► fast-release energy bars
► honey

• Take supplements: (available at most drug, natural food and vitamin stores)
   ► multi vitamin/mineral (see Resource Directory at the end of this book)
   ► brain food: flaxseed (available as oil, ground - wheat germ consistency, or capsules)
   ► B-complex vitamin or nutritional yeast supplement
   ► for added energy: licorice herb or unsweetened licorice candy.
   ► trace mineral supplement

➤digestive enzymes when eating cooked foods (if you are prone to digestive upset)

•Avoid foods which may be detrimental to brain function, containing additives such as:
>➤*aspartame sweetener (may cause headache), MSG (a flavor enhancer), hydrolyzed vegetable protein (in soups). All of these are considered excitotoxins that can affect brain function.*

This program does not radically change your normal diet. It is meant to increase your electrolyte base, and reduce consumption of foods that compromise not only your brain's ability to work at peak performance, but also place a toll on our body, particularly on our muscles. Within two weeks, you should notice a difference, hopefully for the better. If you are used to sugar, caffeine and alcohol as a daily regime, you may feel some withdrawal symptoms such as a headache, when you initially reduce your intake. A few extra glasses of mineral water should help to lessen those symptoms.

If you feel comfortable with our program, you may want to read the following chapters carefully. They will give details about the way nutrition affects our ability to concentrate, to control our temper, to facilitate a smooth golf swing and to lower our score.

Chapter 3. The Western diet: fast and familiar; but a potential handicap for your game.

Menu and snack choices offered at golf clubs, bar and grills, diners, drive-thrus and in pro shops seem universally the same: eggs, bagels with cream cheese, donuts, hot dogs, hamburgers, french fries, pizza, chili, stacked sandwiches or grinders, grilled cheese and bacon. In consideration to their patrons who may be on restricted health diets, restaurants will label their offerings "heart healthy", with subtitles such as "low-cal" or "low-fat" meals. These may include such items as salads with cottage cheese, and broiled fish with vegetables. Next, add the beverages: carbonated drinks, beer, iced tea or coffee. Finally, the "carry-ons" for the cart or golf bag, that are found in the vending machines or the beverage carts, offering candy, cookies, chips and gum. Do these foods help you stay under par? The televised pros, who spend a great deal of time on the course greens, are more and more, regimenting their diets by eating vegetables and fruit.

Professional athletes, pro-golfers included, have blood profile work-ups to make certain that they are fueling their bodies and immune systems properly. Pros are eager to extol the benefits of diet regarding their performance. For example, *Gary*

Player in his book, *Fit For Golf,* states that his on-the-course diet consists of a whole wheat bread sandwich with peanut butter, honey, raisins, dried fruit and bananas.[3] While his choice may have many of you grimacing, he is on the right track .

The wild west atmosphere of nutritional "cures" (bran muffins, to name one) is starting to stabilize. Growing numbers of bone fide laboratories are conducting more research into dietary approaches to health. Also, the public, confused about the safety of foods, wants valid documentation. Although physicians, nutritionists and alternative practitioners don't always agree on the interpretation of data, there is a consensus that long established dietary beliefs are changing. These groups are in absolute agreement that maintaining an unhealthy diet can contribute to disease and general health problems.

Carbohydrates, are no longer the only answer for long-term energy.

When fitness experts told you what to eat before an event, they normally stayed away from protein. Although protein is needed to build and repair muscle, carbohydrates have been considered a better source of energy. For example, it was

---

[3] Reprinted with permission of Simon & Schuster, Inc. from FIT FOR GOLF by Gary Player. Copyright© 1995 by Gary Player.

typical for Olympic participants to carbo-load before their events. *Hale Irwin* in his book *Smart Golf,*[4] tells us to eat a high-carbohydrate meal two hours before the game. However, defining the type of carbohydrates consumed is critical. New information shows that *High Glycemic* (see Appendix D) carbohydrates, which can be found in sugar, potatoes, bagels, and alcohol are a relatively poor source of long-term energy. For stamina over several hours, you should select those carbohydrate foods from a list of long-term energy-sustaining *Low Glycemic Index*[5] foods (see Appendix D). A long list of these foods include whole grain or rye bread, pasta, citrus fruit, apples, grapes, peanuts and milk.

A new trend in research regarding high-powered stamina considers the release of fatty acids as an energy source (your fat cells actually have energy catalysts stored in them). If we exercise after a High Glycemic carbohydrate-rich meal or snack, fatty acid release is slowed and energy production is compromised. However, a Low Glycemic carbohydrate food, prior to exercise, helps to stimulate the release of fatty acids. This process increases the body's rate of energy production (ATP), improving

---

[4] Smart Golf, Hale Irwin ©1999 by Hale Irwin, Harper Collins Publishers, Inc.

[5] Glycemic index ranks foods on how they affect our blood sugar levels. This index measures how much your blood sugar increases in the two or three hours after eating.

our stamina, thus shortening recovery time after exercise. It also helps to prevent the stiffness we get in our muscles after a long day of walking the course. In order to boost our levels of fatty acids, we can add foods such as flaxseed to our diet. It can be eaten in a form similar to wheat germ, or found as an ingredient in a number of sport snack bars available today.

Instead of carbohydrates, protein intake from a specific food program may postpone exhaustion, when taken before an athletic undertaking. Since protein and carbohydrates take different times to digest, it is wise not to eat them together. When combined at the same meal, they raise insulin levels more, and further reduce fatty acid release, compromising your energy source. Eating protein after exercise can reduce recovery time.

Sources of protein, such as nuts and soy, are found in many energy bars. Soybeans actually contain 35% protein. Protein sources from meat take a long time to digest. On the golf course, you need to concentrate your energy on your strokes and strategy, and you don't want to share that needed energy with the digestion of your most recent snack or meal. A wise choice is to eat foods that will be out of the stomach when your muscles start working. Additional protein sources to consider are cheese and yogurt, and ingredients found in certain energy bars. Supplements that contain algae, such as spirulina and chlorophyll, and wheat and barley grass can also provide beneficial proteins.

Short-term vs. long-term energy foods.

Medium and High Glycemic Index[6] carbohydrate foods such as bananas, raisins, pineapple, honey, bagels, croissants, boxed cereal and rice cakes are beneficial for quick *short-term* energy needs. Many pros agree that snacks are critical for helping maintain blood sugar which impacts energy, concentration, and motor skills. Better choices to sustain them for a full day of play, are apples, grapes, popcorn, nuts and energy bars containing slow-release ingredients. These are good *long-term* energy substitutes for the sugar-loaded snacks found in vending machines.

Understanding sugar.

The majority of snacks found in vending machines, such as chips, candy and cookies, contain white sugar, glucose, sucrose or high-fructose corn syrup. These sugars not only contribute to weight gain, but they can also create significant energy imbalances. You've probably watched the television commercials where the farm hand hays 20 acres in

---

[6] A high glyemic index is one that rapidly raises blood sugar levels after it is eaten.

10 seconds after he has eaten a candy bar. It is amusing to watch but more than just advertising entertainment, it conveys bad nutritional information. Simply stated, what goes up must come down. The low energy point usually occurs within one to two hours after eating something that contains a large concentration of sugar. This leaves you feeling tired or hungry for another snack that can boost your energy back up (more sugar).

A specific negative effect of sugar is that it creates a mineral deficiency. Raw sugar contains minerals to help digest it. When sugar is refined (as in white sugar), its natural minerals are stripped away. This creates a deficiency in which minerals must be supplied from within the body to digest the sugar. Refined sugars increase the rate at which we excrete calcium (a mineral). Low levels of calcium can create further mineral imbalances resulting in illnesses of the nerves, bones and cranium.

Another side effect of refined sugar is that it arrests the secretion of gastric juices. This causes the stomach to slow down, and reduces its ability to digest foods. Without proper digestion, you will not absorb nutrients needed for optimum performance. If you must have a snack with a high sugar gram count, eat it one to two hours before or after a meal. This will reduce the negative affects on the digestive process.

Not all sweeteners create blood sugar and digestive imbalances. Fructose, oligofructose and an herbal sweetener, stevia, metabolize slower. We refer to these sugars as slow-release carbohydrates, because they are less likely to give you instant energy followed by fatigue an hour or two later as your blood-sugar balance changes. If you are choosing a food or drink that is sweetened, and you need long-term stamina, select products containing these slow-release sugars.

Foods that work for you.

You cannot pick up a magazine today without reading about cholesterol, diabetes, cancer or some other food-related disease. Foods that affect our health can also affect our performance. *Gary Player* in his book, *Golf Begins at 50*, states, "the foods I avoid for the most part, include: fried or fatty foods, such as pork, bacon, butter, cream, sour cream—these can make you fat and take away energy; refined sugar; tea and coffee; "junk" foods such as white bread and pastries; red meat, which is very indigestible; ice cream, desserts, and other sweets.[7]" Remember, his age is past sixty years and he is still competing successfully in the top ten.

---

[7] Reprinted with permission of Simon & Schuster, Inc. from GOLF BEGINS AT 50 by Gary Player. Copyright© 1988 by Gary Player.

Your choice of food impacts directly:
- your capacity to concentrate
- your ability to control the club
- your temper
- your level of stamina

Some examples of food correlations:
- bananas can combat fatigue
- sunflower seeds may cool your temper
- chicken helps increase your concentration
- nuts support your muscles
- yogurt calms your nerves

Of course, it's not just the food, but specific ingredients in the food that achieve these simple results.

- Foods that *improve brain function* are those high in protein such as soy, beans, flax and whey along with whole grains (rye, millet, whole wheat, spelt, brown rice), and fresh fruit.

- Vegetables that *reduce temper outbursts* by inducing a calming effect, include cauliflower, broccoli and spinach .

- *Stress-reducers* (due to their high vitamin B content) are nuts, seeds, peanuts, fish and bananas.

- When golfers need to *improve performance and overall muscle stamina*, they should increase their protein intake. Protein plays an essential role in the production of hormones and new muscle tissue. The RDA for protein is 60mg. per day for adults, although requirements rise with strenuous exercise. Meat is a good source of protein, but if you have been instructed to limit your fat intake, you may consider other high-protein foods such as flax, wheat and barley grass[8] drinks (see footnote for amounts) and whey.

As a complete protein, flax helps build muscles, blood, internal organs, skin, hair, heart and the brain. It has complex carbohydrates that give us instant calories for energy, as well as regulating our fat metabolism. As an animal protein alternative, wheat and barley grasses also contain lots of vitamin C and bioflavonoids that can slow down cellular aging. Another non-meat source of protein, whey, is found in many sports drinks. For golfers who are lactose intolerant (inability to digest milk sugars), there are some sports drinks that have had the lactose and fat removed from the whey protein.

• Drinking fluids, whether it be a sport's drink or bottled water, is essential for *sustaining maximum concentration and muscle coordination* during the game. In the following chapter, we will investigate the ingredients in several snack products

---

[8] Wheat and barley grass extracts (juice or powder) actually contain 25% protein whereas milk is 3%, eggs 12%, and steak is 16%.

so you can make better choices, depending on the results you desire. results you desire.

Quick reference notes:

► Many physicians, nutritionists and alternative practitioners are changing their ideas about nutrition.

► Gary Player, who in his book, *Fit For Golf* mentions that his on-the-course diet consists of a whole wheat bread sandwich with peanut butter, honey, bananas, raisins and dried fruit. These are a combination of both short and long-term energy foods.

► Carbohydrate foods such as whole grain breads, bananas, raisins, pineapple, honey, and rice cakes are for quick *short-term* energy needs.

► Fatty acids converted from the fats in our body are better for energy production (ATP).

► Snack food choices should have reduced sugar content.

► Power drinks with too much added sugar can cause a rise and fall in one's blood sugar; a short burst of energy followed by fatigue.

► Foods that improve brain function: soy, beans, flax and whey along with whole grains (rye, millet, whole wheat, spelt, brown rice), and fresh fruit.

► Cauliflower, broccoli and spinach can induce a calming effect that reduces temper outbursts.

► Stress-reducers (due to their high vitamin B content) are nuts, seeds, peanuts, fish and bananas.

Chapter 4. Italians are on the right track.

Researchers have studied the Mediterranean diet of wine, pasta and olive oil. They conclude that the benefits derived from this particular diet (antioxidants from grapes, for example), contribute to the health and longevity of these people.

Western diets typically center on fast foods, such as high-fat burgers with super-sized deep-fried potatoes. The traditional Italian meal combines foods that interact beneficially (digestive compatibility) making them much healthier. When eaten together, foods like hamburgers and fries, create digestive imbalance, which contribute to the loss of nutrients. One side effect is a gassy, bloated stomach.

If you are just eating to satisfy your taste buds, this meal will work, but if you want to stay healthy and fit while playing golf, you may want to make another lunch or dinner choice. Wonderful tasting olive-oil-drenched Italian bread, salads with olive oil and vinegar dressing with flaxseed sprinkled on top, and olive oil-based pesto (basil, garlic and parsley) on your spaghetti are better for your health and your game.

Flaxseed contains essential fatty acids (EFAs) which promote recovery from stress, increase mental clarity and calmness, improve learning ability, and increase energy and stamina. Signs of potential deficiencies in EFAs (regarded as the good fats) include:

•brittle nails •dry skin •hair loss •depression •chronic pain •arthritis •migraines •memory loss.

EFAs are also found in fish-liver oil. Research is pointing towards EFAs as a preventive factor in heart disease, because they thin the blood and remove cholesterol. They also have a positive effect on the immune system. A good concentration of EFAs in the body also can contribute to the reduction of a tell-tale sign of aging,—wrinkles.

Essential fats should not be eliminated if you are on a low-fat diet. The brain is 60% fat, and depends on dietary fat for its operation. By restricting all fats for treating certain illness, you may help lower your cholesterol levels. Unfortunately, this also may inhibit your ability to think, by reducing fat levels in the brain. Fats are important to our nerve fibers, but not all fats provide benefit to the body.

Golfers whose diets include a significant amount of fried foods, snack foods and fast foods, may be eating fats that harm their bodies. These foods may contain hydrogenated oils (read those labels) which, when eaten, turn into trans-fats, (known to block arteries, and clog hair follicles which can contribute to baldness). Additional research has found than penile arteries are subjected to the same clogging as heart arteries. Men, if you snack excessively and frequently on pretzels and potato chips containing hydrogenated oil, you may be a candidate for Viagra or one of the many natural alternatives.

Choosing the right fat food.

Olive oil, as previously stated, is a great choice for healthy fats. Perhaps a new food to some of you is flaxseed, which balances the specific type of EFA prevalent in olive oil. Both should be part of your daily diet. Health food stores, mail order food catalogs and gourmet shops carry flaxseed. The appearance of flaxseed is similar to wheat germ. You can find it as an ingredient in a snack bar, which is convenient to take in your snack pack on the course. Flax can aid your brain during critical moments of intense concentration, such as putting.

Butter is also preferred to the choice of margarines that contain hydrogenated oils—again read those labels! If your need for snack foods such as chips, cookies, crackers, and candy, are an essential "comfort food" that you can't be without, there are now many taste-satisfying brands available without hydrogenated oil as an ingredient. These can be found at health food and gourmet stores, and even in some supermarkets.

Taking fat off.

Many take to the golf course to keep fit and stay trim. If you are concerned about your weight, there are several types of fat-blockers available. These work by preventing the digestion (and subsequent absorption) of fat. Fat blockers can have adverse side-effects; therefore, it would be prudent to consult a health practitioner prior to undertaking any fat-blocking regime.

One of the safest fat blockers is an ingredient in the spring-harvested Rhododendron caucasicum plant. Discovered in the high mountains of the Georgian republic of the former USSR, a constituent in this herb has the ability to inhibit lipase (the enzyme responsible for fat digestion). By not being digested, the fat is unable to pass through the intestinal wall. This prevents absorption and accumulation in your thighs or belly. Possibly because of the herb's strong medicinal qualities, these Georgians live to be 120 years old. Preventing weight gain with this herb does not affect essential fatty acid absorption.

A key to fat reduction comes from using up the fat, and not from speeding up your metabolism, a belief which has long been held by many dieters. Obviously, by eating less, you can reduce body mass as long as you exercise during the diet. Even if you jog to the next tee instead of riding in the cart, many find that fat remains. A contributing factor is the body's lack of sufficient levels of a specific enzyme (lipase), that releases the fat from the fat parts of the body and converts it into fatty acids used for ATP production. ATP is what gives us energy when we exercise, and by burning this fat, we eliminate it from the body. Fats not broken down will result in the depletion of ATP during exercise, causing fatigue and a slow recovery rate. Therefore, it is necessary to have medical personnel determine if your lipase levels are adequate for fat breakdown. If you discover a deficiency, you may want to add supplemental enzymes to your diet.

Choosing Fat-reducing products.

Rhododendron caucasicum is widely distributed in health food stores as well as pharmacies and through multi-level-marketing companies which are networking companies. As with any fat-blocker, contact your health practitioner to see if it is appropriate for your condition. The herbal supplement, Rhodiola rosea, is another herb useful for weight control. It is an effective fat-releaser and has been clinically proven to be extremely effective in weight loss programs. Supplements can be purchased at health food stores, pharmacies, herbal weight loss clinics and through multi-level-marketing companies. The enzyme lipase is available as a supplement although many products also include other types of enzymes. Remember that fat-releasers only work if you exercise and "burn" the fat converted into fatty acids.

Quick reference notes:
►The good fats reduce stress, and increase mental clarity, learning ability, energy and stamina, and help keep you calm, cool and collected.
►Good fats (EFAs) come from flaxseed and fish liver oils.
►Low-fat diets may inhibit your ability to think, by reducing necessary fat levels in the brain.
►Hydrogenated oils, found in most snack foods, when eaten, turn into trans-fats, (goo which blocks arteries and clogs hair follicles contributing to baldness)

Chapter 5. Snack Bars and Sports Drinks, choosing the right one for you.

The most important ingredient needed in sports drinks is electrolytes (refer back to Chapter 1), for their extremely vital minerals. To re-hydrate the body, many sports drinks add electrolytes and carbohydrates, both of which increase fluid uptake from the intestines into the bloodstream. Research shows that the body absorbs more fluid when electrolytes are added. Some sports drinks provide a more *balanced* base of electrolytes by including potassium, sodium, copper, iodine, manganese, zinc, selenium, and chromium. Providing a combination of electrolytes guards against a mineral imbalance in the body. This can occur when an excess of a single mineral tries to maintain balance by depleting stores of other minerals .

Sports drinks also include carbohydrates in the form of a sweetener (sucrose, glucose, high-fructose corn syrup). Research from the American College of Sports Medicine shows that carbohydrates increase water absorption by interacting with sodium, which is stimulated by glucose. The advantage of this school of thought is that the quicker we ingest carbohydrates after exercise, the quicker we will replace muscle glycogen.[9] The downside is that simple carbohydrates in the form of sugar can put our blood sugar on a roller-coaster ride, which reduces the long-term energy-producing benefits of the drink. In an effort to offer an alternative to regular sugar, several companies are adding rice syrup, which is 60% complex carbohydrate, but less than 15 % simple sugars or oligofructose (a slow-release sugar). These sweeteners are metabolized steadily and offer an even source of energy.

In the pages that follow, you will find a comparison chart of the most popular sports drinks and energy bars. The ingredients listed are only a representative sample, and may not include a complete representation of the product. However, this list will give you enough data to determine which products can maintain long-term stamina, or those you would purchase for short-term energy boosts. We also have detailed unfamiliar ingredients, and those that may not promote health.

---

[9] Glycogen metabolizes into glucose molecules and fuels the body during moderate exercise.

Sports drink comparison.

Brand	Calories	Sodium	Potassium	Carbos	Sugars
Dasani	0	0g	0mg	0g	0g
Gatorade	50	110mg	30mg	14g	14g
Golf Lyte	0	0mg	0mg	0g	0g
Golf Pro	65	0mg	25mg	17g	17g
Hy-Lytes	50	0g	36.2mg	13g	13g
Perform	60	1.10mg	35mg	16g	13g
Powerade	70	55mg	30mg	19g	15g
Pro-Energizer	400	40mg	77mg	100g	n/a
Snapple Hydro	100	40mg	0mg	24g	23g
Ultima	40	20mg	39mg	10g	0g

Brand	Primary ingredients, in addition to water
Dasani	magnesium sulfate, potassium chloride, salt (negligible)
Gatorade	sucrose, dextrose, citric acid, natural flavors, salt, partially hydrogenated coconut oil, yellow 5 lake, yellow 6 lake.
Golf Lyte	11 trace minerals, MSM, vitamin C
Golf Pro	ginkgo biloba herb, choline, ginseng, vitamin B_{12}
Hy-Lytes (powder mix)	Dry fructose, citric acid, calcium aspartate, glycine, potassium aspartate, manganese aspartate, magnesium aspartate, chromium aspartate, selenium aspartate
Perform	glucose, crystalline fructose, sodium citrate, monopotassium phosphate,
Powerade	high fructose corn syrup, maltodextrin, potassium citrate, salt, acacia, potassium phosphate, coconut oil, blue 1
Pro Energizer	glucose polymers, fructose, high fructose corn syrup, fruit juices, potassium phosphate, FD&C red #40
Snapple Hydro	high fructose corn syrup, pear juice, beta carotene, salt
Ultima	70 ionic minerals, grape seed, pantothenic acid, CoQ_{10}, maltodextrin, potassium citrate, magnesium aspartate, stevia

General analysis of ingredients:

•FD & C Red #40, Yellow 5 and 6: dyes that are suspected potential carcinogens. Yellow 5 lake refers to a combination of FD & C colors with a form of aluminum or calcium which makes them insoluble.

•Grams of sugars indicated in drinks related to total sugars (from natural ingredients as well as added sweeteners)

•Maltodextrin (fast-release) is sugar obtained by the hydrolysis of starch and is used as a texturizer and flavor enhancer.

•MSM: an organic crystalline compound that comprises 34% elemental sulfur, beneficial for certain conditions (see Appendix A).

•Vitamin B12 is known as the "pep vitamin" and supports proper nerve transmission.

•Hydrogenated or partially hydrogenated oil: This ingredient is suspected in raising blood cholesterol. The American Heart Association in their online website[10] recommends looking for processed foods made with <u>un</u>hydrogenated oil rather than hydrogenated, or saturated fat. This means that you had better take up label-reading when you go shopping.

---

[10] Reproduced with permission American Heart Association World Wide Web Site: www.americanheart.org/Heart_and_Stroke_A_Z_Guide/tfa.html, 1998 Copyright American Heart Association

- Sweeteners:

Quick release:

Glucose: a crystalline sugar

Sucrose: sugar from sugar cane

Dextrose: a glucose sugar

High fructose corn syrup is commercial glucose (sugar) from chemically purified cornstarch.

Slow-release:

Fructose: a crystalline sugar found in sweet fruits and in honey.

Oligofructose: a nondigestible fiber carbohydrate sweetener with slow-release properties.

Stevia: an herbal sweetener, is 25 times sweeter than table sugar.

Grape and pear juice: natural sweeteners which provide simple carbohydrates for energy.

Brown rice syrup: a mild sweetener that offers a slower complex carbohydrate release that has good staying power.

Sports bar comparison.

Energy bars that are finding their way into pro shops and on snack carts, are a welcome substitute for a candy bar. Not all energy bars are created equal. Many contain large quantities of sugar that give you a quick burst of energy, but little staying power for 18 holes of golf. And, just like candy bars, flavor drives most decisions in selection (ah, that sugar again). Try to remember however, with a little practice you can acquire a taste for many things you once thought unimaginable, especially if you know they are partners with you in maintaining good health.

Brand	Calories	Protein	Fat	Carbos	Sugar
Balance	200	22g	5g	17g	13g
Breakthru	220	12g	3g	37g	16g
Clif	250	4g	3g	51g	14g
Flaxeon	220	22g	8g	32g	3g
Golf Pro	205	4.5g	3g	40g	15g
Iron Man	230	16g	8g	24g	16g
Luna women's	170	10g	3g	26g	12g
Mountain Lift	220	12g	4.5g	33g	20g
Omega Bar	168	5.3g	4.42g	25g	n/a
Power Bar Harvest	240	7g	4g	45g	18g
Power Bar	230	10g	2.5 g	45g	18g
Stealth	230	9g	6g	37g	25g
Think	205	4.5g	3g	40g	15g

Brand	Primary ingredients, in addition to water
Balance Bar	soy protein, whey protein, high fructose corn syrup, honey, sugar, ground peanuts, palm kernel oil, nonfat milk, nonfat yogurt, salt, dextrose, lecithin, chicory, oligofructose, vitamins, minerals
Breakthru	soy protein, raisins, malted cereal syrup, oats, cashews, minerals, soybeans, flax, evaporated cane juice, herbs, vitamins, bioflavonoids, sea vegetables
Clif Bar	Rolled oats, brown rice syrup, grape juice concentrate, beta carotene, rice flour, corn meal, figs, barley malt, cocoa powder, coffee beans, vitamins
Flaxeon	soy protein complex, whey protein, flaxseed, rolled oats, almonds, fructose, rice flour. malt, salt
Golf Pro	fruit, oat bran, rice flour, choline, ginseng, chamomile, gingko
Iron Man	soy, whey, high fructose corn syrup, peanut butter, sucrose, yogurt solids, non-fat dry milk, lecithin, vitamins, minerals, biotin
Luna	brown rice syrup, soy, rice, rolled oats, raisins, cashews, almonds, lecithin, green tea, minerals, pumpkin seeds
Mountain Lift	soy protein, ginseng, ginkgo biloba, 12 essential vitamins
Omega Bar	flax, brown rice syrup, peanut butter, dates, apricots, bananas
Power Bar	high fructose corn syrup with grape and pear juice concentrate, oat bran, maltodextrin, raisins, milk protein, brown rice, vitamins, minerals, amino acids
Power Bar Harvest	whole oats, brown rice syrup, dried strawberries, brown rice, almond butter, roasted soy beans, soy protein concentrate, honey, pear and grape juice concentrates,
Stealth	whey (protein) glucose, fructose, maltodextrin, glucose, sucrose, raisins, honey, soy lecithin, bilberry, gingko, Siberian ginseng, Canadian ginseng, vitamins, minerals
Think	rice syrup, oat bran, rice flour, rolled oats, oat bran, almond butter, brown rice, gingko, ginseng, chamomile

Short-term energy ingredients: high fructose corn syrup, honey, sugar, maltodextrin, dextrose, cane juice, raisins, corn meal, bananas.

Long-term energy ingredients: brown rice syrup, soy, whey, peanuts, flax, oats, barley, brown rice, milk, grape juice, pear juice, yogurt, oligofructose.

How to determine if an energy bar provides slow or fast-release of nutrients:
a) read the label on your selected energy bar or refer to the comparison chart on page 49.
b) refer to page 47 and determine the specific type of sweetener included in the bar.
c) refer to Appendix D to determine the High Glycemic (fast-release) or Low Glycemic (slow-release) ingredients contained in the bar.

Note: Slow-release energy bars referred to in the TEE TIME DIET are for long term stamina. Quick or fast-release energy bars are for short bursts of energy. They should be followed by a food from the Low Gycemic chart in Appendix D within 1-2 hours to prevent blood sugar imbalances and associated symptoms (fatigue and/or food cravings as an example).

Chapter 6. Leverage your game: smart food and beverage choices.

The snacks, beverages and meals suggested in this chapter are based on common factors for all people. It is acknowledged that different people tolerate foods in different ways. Onions and garlic can create a love or hate relationship with eaters. Tomatoes can crown pasta meals, or bring about extreme allergic reactions. Each of us is different, and by adulthood you know which foods you need to avoid.

For those of you who do not walk the course, and ride a cart instead, we advise that you follow the same menu, cutting the quantity you eat by one-third. This diet is meant for the day of play only. It is not meant as a permanent lifestyle change, nor should it be followed if your physician has prescribed a specific dietary consideration for a medical condition.

Today, the majority of pro golfers are very conscious of their diets, and not because they're concerned about looking fit and trim on television. Their diets and supplements vary, but their motivation is the same; supporting their bodies and brain through smart eating, to increase their potential to win. *Dr. Deborah Graham, Ph.D.* sports psychologist for hundreds of PGA, Sr. PGA, LPGA and Nike Tour players and co-author of *The*

8 Traits of Champion Golfers says, "You burn a tremendous number of calories in a round of golf. For this reason you need to eat a well-balanced meal before the round and to take nutritious snacks on the course. These snacks are even more important for the person who is too nervous to eat well before the round."

Some example of pros choosing nutritional avenues: *Jesper Parnevik* advocates vitamins, producing his own line of supplements. *Bob Charles,* a former British Open champion, uses deer antler velvet supplements along with shark cartilage to promote longevity. *Jose Maria Olazabal* attributes his recovery from podiatry problems to shark cartilage extract, glucosamine, chondroitin, vitamins, minerals and specific polyunsaturated fatty acids.

Recommendations—Background.

Proteins are needed to improve stamina. Since protein plays an essential role in the production of hormones and new muscle tissue, it is important to maintain adequate stores. Golfers call upon muscle tissue to provide adequate ball control, and stamina, to walk the 18 holes. Therefore, a protein meal should be included early in the day.

Prior to teeing off, a long-term energy carbohydrate food would give a boost to get you going. Snacks on the course should be structured again for long-term stamina. Any short-term energy foods eaten for a quick burst during a demanding hole, should be followed by a long-term carbohydrate food within one half-hour to prevent a blood sugar low, and resultant fatigue.

We have structured a list of suggested foods for maintaining high performance levels, depending on the time of play. These will give you the leverage you need for maximizing your power of concentration, and also for strong, accurate muscle delivery.

This plan is based on maintaining your energy at an even level. Sustaining adequate carbohydrate levels by eating a slow-release Low Glycemic food during play regardless of your appetite, will prevent radical blood sugar highs or lows. After the game, you can choose carbohydrate foods that have a High Glycemic Index (fast-release), which can provide a quicker recovery from stressed muscles. These should be followed by a Low-Glycemic Index carbohydrate (slow-release) before the blood sugar swing starts affecting your ability to stay awake on the drive home. According to Dr. Uma Viswanathan, "watching your blood sugar is just as important as watching your score card. If you eat sensibly, you can improve your stamina and concentration and have a great game of golf."

TEE TIME DIET

This diet was constructed in collaboration with Dr. Uma Viswanathan, M.D., C.C.N., who practices in Ridgefield, CT. and Neil Orenstein, Ph.D., formerly affiliated with the Massachusetts General Hospital and Beth Israel Hospital (Harvard Medical School) in Boston.

<u>TEE TIMES: SUNRISE TO 10:30 A.M.</u>

Wake-up:
•Get in the habit of drinking a glass of water upon rising. The best is mineral water (bottled or water with liquid supplements added). Water with extra minerals acts as a cleanser and provides the electrolytes to "charge" the brain.

Breakfast:
Eat at least two hours before playing
•*Food:* eggs, turkey bacon or turkey sausage (less fat), beef, smoked salmon (unless you're on a salt restricted diet), fish, oatmeal.
• *Beverage*: mineral water, whey or soy powder drink (without sugar added–fructose OK), unsweetened fruit juice. *Coffee/Tea:* For maximum performance try to avoid caffeinated beverages on the day of play. If you must have that "wake-up"

54

cup, follow it with a chaser of purified water. Refrain from adding sugar on the day of play.

Supplements for extra boost:
Multi-vitamin, flax capsule or powder, lecithin capsule, digestive enzyme (with breakfast) for added absorption of nutrients.
For extra oomph, barley or wheat grass (tablet or juice), alfalfa tablets (prevents exhaustion).
Choose additional supplements from Appendix A, depending on your needs.

Just before teeing off:
•*Food*: Maintain carbohydrate levels by eating a slow-release carbohydrate such as a slice of rye toast or oat bran muffin (no white breads), a bowl of whole grain cereal (no sugar added), slow-release energy bar or citrus fruit like an orange or grapefruit.
• *Beverage:* another glass of mineral water.

Snacks to travel the course:
Mandatory: A *big* bottle of purified water.
Optional:
Food: apples, grapes, sunflower seeds (high in potassium), nuts, celery sticks, granola (no sugar added), sports bar (slow release ingredients).

Beverage: In addition to water: <u>unsweetened </u>cran-berry, apple, lemon, or citrus juice.

After The First Nine:
Food: dark flour bread or muffins (no white bread, corn muffins, bagels or donuts) *or*
slow-release energy sports bar *or*
apple, plum, tomato, peach.
Soups: tomato, lentil or vegetable soup, (if the weather is cold and the course has them available).
Beverage: more mineral water or unsweetened fruit juices, unsweetened electrolyte drink.
Note: if you break for lunch, select slow release carbohydrates such as tuna or peanut butter sand-wich, yogurt, chili or salad.

Last Nine Holes:
Food: Slow-release energy bar, nuts *or*
sunflower seeds, apple.
Note: Last hour of play, a quick-release food is permitted such as: bananas, raisins, quick-release energy bar.
Beverage: More mineral water or unsweetened fruit juice, unsweetened electrolyte drink.

After the Game: Lunch
Food: To recover from muscle usage, eat a fast-release carbohydrate lunch such as: Bagel,

sandwiches such as beef, chicken, tuna or turkey, salads with chicken, whole milk yogurt, veggie burgers, sardines, potatoes, corn, cheese, tacos. Soups: green pea, squash, chicken.

Beverage: sparkling mineral water, fruit juice, tea or coffee. (Alcohol is not recommended if you are playing another round, going back to work or driving.)

TEE TIME: After 10:30 A.M.

Recommendations are basically similar.
Refer to the lists for earlier tee times for breakfast and snacks to take along.

Change for: At the turn–9 holes down, lunch or extra snack.

Food: Eat a slow-release food such as yogurt (low fat), slow-release energy bar, bean salad, hummus (chick peas), sandwich on dark bread: turkey, tuna, peanut butter. veggie burger, chili.
Soups: tomato or vegetable.

Beverage: iced tea (no sugar), mineral water, unsweetened fruit juices: cranberry, apple, lemonade, or citrus, unsweetened electrolyte drink.

TEE TIME: 1:30 to mid-afternoon
Follow the wake-up, breakfast, and items to pack
for snacks that have already outlined.

Lunch: finish at least 1 hour before start
•_Eat a slow-release carbohydrate meal_ such as:
Salad bar (no white bread); chili; sandwich: turkey,
tuna, peanut or almond butter on dark bread; fet-
tuccini with tomato sauce or pesto; fish, cole slaw,
broccoli, cauliflower, spinach, collards, kale.
Soup: onion, vegetable.
•_Beverage:_ Sparkling water with lemon or lime,
unsweetened fruit juice. (no alcohol or soda pop).
•_Dessert:_ none.

Break: At the turn:
•_Slow-release foods_ such as apple, plum, tomato,
tangerine, celery and zucchini sticks, sunflower
seeds, slow-release energy bar.
•_Beverage:_ mineral water, unsweetened electrolyte
drink or unsweetened juices.

19th Hole "Happy Hour":
•_Food:_ cheese and crackers, nachos, carrot sticks,
bagels, rice cakes, corn chips, nuts.
•_Beverage:_ mineral water, fruit juice or quick release sport's drink, alcohol (in moderation).

TEE TIME: Late Afternoon, Early Evening

•Follow the recommended choices for wake-up, breakfast and lunch.

•Drink lots of mineral water throughout the day.

•If you must drink coffee, make certain that you finish it 1 hour before teeing off and follow each cup with a chaser of purified water.

•If you are playing with only a minimal break to get in a few more holes, or race the darkness for 18 holes, take along plenty of the snacks listed.

•Happy Hour overlaps this time frame. Try to avoid consuming any alcohol before you finish for the day, and refrain from snacking on fast-release foods.

If You are Playing Two Days in a Row

•_Dinner Recommendations_

Note: Allow one hour after happy hour to give fast-release foods time to digest and remove sugars from stomach.

•_Food:_ slow-release energy food such as: pasta: with meatless tomato sauce or pesto, salad, meatless lasagna, vegetables, beans, rice, fish, peas, asparagus, broccoli, cauliflower, sweet potatoes.

•_Beverage:_ mineral water, herbal tea, slow-energy sports drink. _Note: If you are used to consuming alcohol at dinner, limit it to a glass of wine, rather than high-sugar hard liquor._

•_Dessert:_ none

After the game, it is important to put back nutrients that are used up due to exercise, stress or mental strain. Water is the number one replacement item because rehydration is extremely important to facilitate restoration of muscle tone and bodily function. Exercise can make us lose the equivalent of 1½ gallons of water through sweat. For example, marathon runners metabolize about ¾ pound of fat, but lose up to ten pounds of water weight.

Drinks with added electrolytes are a good choice. Electrolytes facilitate the removal of lactic acid build-up in the muscles, which contributes to the soreness and stiffness we feel the day after our workout. Some drinks also have added sodium and carbohydrates, which increases fluid uptake from the intestines into the bloodstream.

Fast-release carbohydrate meals may be important as a post-exercise (physical) regime. If muscle glycogen is used up during exercise, it must be replaced. High Glycemic Index carbohydrates assist in this process, and therefore should be eaten shortly *after* exercise. Many diets recommend eating sugar to replace glycogen. Although it does seem to help muscle glycogen to recover faster, it may place an overall toll on your body. This is because of the blood sugar imbalances it causes. It also adds to the storage of fat in your body. Therefore, follow our recommendations in the Tee Time Diet for late-day meals, and avoid a lot of high-sugar carbohydrate replacement foods and drink.

One of the key factors in recovery and maintaining a high energy level is to produce more energy-containing molecules, referred to as ATP (adenosine triphosphate) and Creatine phosphate. ATP is generated by the oxidation of carbohydrates, fat and protein, and is used up in great quantities during exercise. It needs to be constantly replenished, and depends on the burning of fatty acids and glycogen for this process. Creatine helps to maintain ATP levels.

The herb, Rhodiola rosea, has been shown to increase muscle ATP and creatine levels, and increase the fatty acids in the blood. Adding Rhodiola rosea herbal supplement *before* exercise, positively changes the protein balance in athletes, and increases the mass of contractile muscle fibers during workout. This results in a reduction in the duration of the recovery period. In experiments with 112 athletes, 89% of those receiving Rhodiola extract showed less fatigue after exercise, less muscle stiffness, and a quicker recovery from the stress of exercise.

SECTION 2. HUMAN FACTORS

Chapter 8. Temper and Mental acuity.

Numerous books have been written on the mental aspect of golf. Focus, concentration, visualization and a positive attitude all play a large part in how you score. Proper mental techniques work. These methods will work even better if you support your brain chemistry by supplementing your diet with amino acids, lecithin or flax.

Knowing how to sink an easy putt, and actually getting it into the cup, depend on a close relationship between mind and muscle. If the mind is shooting erroneous signals due to a chemical breakdown, you may lose control of the muscle in your arm. This results in the ball ending up somewhere other than the intended cup. The chemical breakdown in the brain will then cause you to throw your putter, and utter unintelligible words often referencing "god and mother".

Most advice we have received regarding controlling our temper has come from psychologists. Often they tell us to slowly count to 10 and recognize that "acting out" is not an effective way to vent anger. The idea that catharsis is the best way to handle anger is no longer accepted by researchers.

Studies have discovered that venting anger by pounding the ground with your club or tossing it past the caddie, increases rather than decreases further aggressive behavior.[11] *Dr. Deborah Graham, Ph.D.,* a psychologist working full time with PGA, Sr. PGA, LPGA and Nike Tour players states, "Anxiety or tension can be increased and decreased by the foods we eat. Certain foods and nutritional supplements can help calm us. Other foods can create increased tension. You need to become more aware of the effects of the foods and supplements you eat to manage this possible source of increasing tension and anxiety."

Analyzing behavior anomalies without addressing the chemical breakdowns in the brain caused by nutritional deficiencies, is putting the cart before the horse. The messages creating emotions are transmitted between cells in the human brain by neurotransmitters. Neurotransmitter deficiencies caused by diets low in amino acids, through genetics, stress, as well as alcohol and/or drug abuse can short circuit these message pathways.

Temper outbursts can happen at the least provocation. You may also feel depressed, lethargic, moody, irritable, and anxious; experience sleeplessness, food cravings and addictions.

[11] Extracted from studies appearing in The Journal of Personality and Social Psychology, March, 1999

Depleted supplies of the feel-good neuro-transmitters (endorphins) make it difficult for you to feel happy, on track and motivated. Muscle control and accuracy can also be affected by deficiencies in specific amino acids.

Supplementing your diet with flaxseed and lecithin can support the operation of nerve fibers in the brain. Lecithin, used as an emulsifier in many foods, is necessary for the smooth flow of messages through the nervous system, thereby preventing disruption of muscle coordination. The essential fatty acids (EFAs) in flax, aid the transmission of nerve impulses that are needed for normal brain functioning.

Brain-enhancing herbs are also finding their way into power-bars and sports drinks. Gingko biloba is purported to increase mental alertness; kava kava and ginger work together to act as a re-laxant to control temper; Maca, a Peruvian herb, promotes mental clarity and camu-camu is used to control anxiety. Rhodiola rosea herbal extract has been shown to influence learning and memory by supporting neurotransmitters and affecting brain chemistry. Tests using Rhodiola showed that it effectively improved coordination. Rosemary, which can be added to your bath, can help relieve bouts of depression, mental fatigue, lethargy or apathy after a poor game. Sage has a natural ability to feed the nerves, so it is useful after a temper outburst. It also supplies oxygen to the cortex of the brain, which acts to revitalize it and bring thoughts into better focus.

According to Dr. Deborah Graham and Jon Stabler who wrote, *The 8 Traits of Champion Golfers,* [12] "Everyone's body chemistry is different, and has a direct impact on the way we experience emotions. If you work hard to change your thoughts and attitudes, but cannot modify your emotional reactions, you may need to look more closely for biological reasons. A change in diet, increasing exercise levels, using certain supplements, and possibly an anti-depressant medication, may help you gain increased control over your emotions when your biology is a contributor to mental stress."

Some of the effects on our brain actually come from our body. Golfers put their muscles through some rather extraordinary trauma. Repeated swings to one side, constant bending and twisting and playing without stretching first, can all lock up our muscles, restricting nerve impulses to the brain resulting in tension, anxiety, restlessness and irritability. Supplements, or brain-supporting foods may help, but to effect long term benefits, focus should

---

[12] *The 8 Traits of Champion Golfers,* (888) 280-4653

be given to correcting the underlying problem. Our next chapter will discuss some not-so-familiar treatments for back pain and muscle trauma.

Choosing a brain supplement.

Amino acids from meat, eggs and dairy sources are essential as protein sources for the body. Lecithin is an excellent addition to your morning supplement regime. Flaxseed is available at most health food stores as a condiment, or in supplement form. For snacking on the course, you can also purchase an energy bar with flax as an ingredient.

Herbs that are used for brain power can be found in power bars and power drinks, as well as supplements and herbal tinctures. Most are available through health food stores, pharmacies and mail order. You can make your own herbal concoctions if you are so inclined, by mixing herbal essential oils with a base oil such as apricot kernel oil or peanut oil. More on this process can be found in the book *Plant Power*, by herbalist Laurel Dewey (see Recommended Reading list).

Chapter 9. Aching backs, stiff joints and muscle fatigue.

Fitness experts always recommend that before exercise, you should include some preconditioning, such as stretching. Since many of us go from car to cart to course without stretching, the repeated twisting motion from swinging the clubs or climbing up a steep bunker or embankment can contribute to traumatized extremities, if we don't warm up. Difficult terrains cause a number of problems for our muscles. Tiger Woods while playing in the 1999 British Open at Carnoustie was quoted, "you could seriously injure yourself in this rough, and you are always going to get worn out." (New York Post July 16, 1999) .

Suffering from a tight muscle can make your body compensate with a limp or a neck crook. The result we most often feel from these traumas is real pain manifested in our back, shoulders, wrists and legs. Stretching and sticking to a regime of exercise protects back muscles and your back, and will reduce your risk of injury no matter what type of course you play on.

Our back, the most frequent golf casualty.

The Classic golf swing follow-through has the body in an "I" position. If you have switched to the form that mocks a reverse C, you may be getting extra distance on the ball, but you are adding stress on the body, and compounding the risk of back and muscle problems. Repetitive motion causes muscles and joints to compensate, when the movement is exclusively right handed or left-handed. This imbalance can create back pain as well as muscle aches from overuse.

By the time chronic pain settles in, one usually seeks medical help. Doctors prescribe pain killers more often than not, such as aspirin or more powerful prescriptions, and advise that you take it easy. This course of action can relieve pain temporarily, but seldom fixes the underlying problem. Chronic back pain may require surgery. However, in some conditions the doctors will first refer you to a physical therapist. There are "alternative" methods of treatment available as well to consider. They include massage therapy, chiropractic adjustments, Myofascial muscle release and CranioSacral treatments. The last two may be new to you, but know that a large number of qualified practitioners are available all over the United States. Many professional golfers use at least one of these methods to help reduce tension and pain.

Nutritional support for back pain:

•Drink at least eight glasses of water per day. Chronic dehydration can actually result in back pain. Drinking lots of water also flushes acid particles from the system, to support proper kidney function.

•Avoid foods that contain high levels of uric acid which can aggravate back pain, such as: red meats, pasteurized dairy products, and caffeine.

• Your diet should be high in minerals and vegetable proteins, with a focus on reduction of fats (see Chapter 4). *Note: Carrying excess weight can contribute to back pain. Therefore, a weight loss program may be advised.*

•Herbal remedies for consideration:

　►Rhodiola rosea builds resistance to fatigue, enhances back muscle strength and hand-strength endurance.

　►Rosemary herbal cream for sore muscles.

　►Thyme rub-on application for inflammation caused by sprains.

　► Skullcap (taken orally) known to be effective to take the edge off the pain.

•For additional consideration, refer to supplements which are discussed in Chapter 13.

Muscles and joints.

Muscle support is necessary for accurate ball control. When our joints and muscles ache, our performance is compromised, and instead of looking forward to the 19th hole, we look forward to just grabbing a comfortable place to lie or sit down. Again we repeat, stretching and warm-ups can reduce stress on our muscles. Muscle and joint challenges from golf can include some of the following:

►Walking a course with varied terrain may cause cramping in the calf, feet and leg.

►The swinging motion of the arm can cause Golfer's elbow, an inflammation of the muscles in the forearm and tendons which are connected to the elbow.

►The way you repeatedly grip your clubs can create thumb tendonitis.

►Seniors who tend to use a more upright stance develop neck pain as they reduce the forward thrust of their head during the swing.

►Muscle pain is frequently caused by a twist, turn, chronic neck position or trauma to the body. Other parts of the body can be affected, producing pain somewhere else. A certified practitioner can properly identify all the muscles and joints involved in the injury, effecting a course of treatment for the root cause, rather than just reducing pain in the specific spot of discomfort.

►Thinking can be affected by muscle stress. Tense muscles can create nerve restriction up the spine. This may affect neural signals to the brain affecting emotions and thinking ability. In other words; it's difficult to concentrate on your game when your body hurts. Dr. John Upledger, from the Upledger Institute in Palm Beach Gardens, Florida, finds that when our bodies compensate for injuries, symptoms such as headaches, dizziness or vertigo can manifest. This can be nothing more than the membrane system surrounding the brain reacting to a body that is out of alignment.

►Joints can be affected by repetitive motion, and also by an arthritic buildup of waste particles. Adequate mineral stores can facilitate moving these particles from the joints, and flushing them from the body.

Muscle chemistry.

Much stiffness and muscular immobility comes after long strenuous exercise. To understand why this happens, we will describe the process that your body undertakes to make the muscles work. Glycogen is an energy source produced and stored in muscle tissue. During exercise, a catabolic hormone, cortisol, is secreted, that stimulates glucose production necessary for quick mental and physical reactions. When our normal levels of ATP *(see*

Chapter 4) are diminished, and exercise is prolonged, the body turns to the muscle for fuel, by changing the glycogen into the simple sugar, glucose. Vitamin C also increases the amount of glycogen stored in muscle tissue.

To prevent using up glycogen stores, we can look for another source of ATP, the fatty acids from body fat. As discussed previously, fats that are not broken down will result in the depletion of ATP during exercise, resulting in greater muscle fatigue and a slower recovery rate.

One can consider supporting the body by taking supplemental lipase enzymes (to break down the fats). You can also use the herb, Rhodiola rosea to release fatty acids from the fat, to boost available stores of ATP and reduce the usage of glycogen, thus reducing the need to carbo-load after exercise, to replace lost glycogen.

Nutritional support recommendations for muscle and joint stiffness:
• Water is an absolute necessity for proper muscular action. Dehydration has a negative effect on muscle operation, but also can reduce potassium levels. A loss of this essential element results in muscle weakness. For preventive care, you should drink mineral water, as the electrolytes facilitate the removal of lactic acid build-up in the muscles. This

74

build-up contributes to the soreness and stiffness we feel the day after we have played 18 holes.

• Deficiencies of sulfur, an essential mineral, also can contribute to muscle pain. Foods containing sulfur such as milk, beans, garlic, onions, wheat germ, fresh fruit, eggs, meat and seafood contain MSM, an organic crystalline compound that comprises 34% elemental sulfur. Brittle hair and nails, arthritis, acne and depression are common indications of sulfur deficiency.

Fortunately, MSM is also available as a topical or oral supplement, and has been widely used to treat muscle and joint pain, particularly when the joint is breaking down. Scientists have discovered that people with damaged cartilage have 1/3 lower sulfur levels than people with normal tissue. MSM deficiencies have been linked to osteoarthritis and rheumatoid arthritis. MSM supplementation may help to reduce muscle and joint pain, as it acts as a muscle relaxant.

•Supplementation with the enzyme lipase and the herb, Rhodiola rosea (capsule), help to prevent ATP depletion and muscle stiffness.

•Lecithin, a fat-like substance, when in adequate supply, can prevent the breakdown of muscle control.

•Glucosamine Sulfate, which keeps joints elastic, and helps to relieve the pain and inflammation of osteoarthritis, is a good alternative to non-steroidal anti-inflammatory drugs, which may have unwanted side effects.

•B_{12} is a "pep" vitamin that helps neuro-muscular control. By building a protein sheath around the nerve fibers, it can reduce symptoms of muscle spasms, prickly sensations in the hands and feet, and unsteadiness.

•Vitamin C increases the amount of glycogen stored in the muscles, which is needed for energy release. When it is depleted, our muscles become stiff and sore. Corticosteroids such as Cortisone and Prednisone may facilitate excretion of vitamin C, as well as potassium and zinc.

•Potassium is needed to convert blood sugar into glycogen for muscle energy. Deficiencies result in muscle weakness and fatigue. You may help to replace potassium by eating potassium-rich foods such as kelp, sunflower seeds, wheat germ, almonds, raisins, parsley, peanuts, dates, avocado, garlic, spinach and beans, to name a few.

•Homeopathic pain relievers such as arnica, hypericum, rhus tox and, ruta graveolens may be considered.

•Herbal ginseng and flower remedies are known to give on-the-spot relief.

•Velvet antler is used as an aphrodisiac and as a treatment for arthritic and joint pain.

Chapter 10. The unwanted visitor: the headache.

Headaches not caused by back, neck and eye strain, may be caused by dehydration, mineral deficiency, hormonal imbalance, allergies or diet, a pulled muscle, hip or knee misalignment. Randi and Jim Haskins, licensed Physical Therapists practicing in Great Barrington, Massachusetts report, "most of the headache-causing dysfunction we see, seems related to abnormal wear patterns in the body, such as shoulder tendonitis. If not addressed, these symptoms may progress to the wrist, neck and jaw, and head. Headache pain is actually the body's cry for help. Treatment should employ therapists who address the cause behind the pain, not just prescribe an ointment or a pill to relieve the pain."

Fixing the cause of the headache is the ultimate corrective procedure, but many times we need instant relief. Whether you choose over-the-counter or natural headache remedies, remember that when your head hurts, it means something is wrong. An occasional headache from dehydration or a hangover can be a nuisance, but chronic and migraine headaches should alert you to a more serious problem needing the care of a health practitioner.

Non-drug treatments for headaches include:

•Bromelain which acts like aspirin without risk of stomach upset.

•Niacin can help to keep the blood vessels and circulation open.

•Oxygen drops (found in health food stores) or a brisk walk can help restore proper oxygen levels in the brain.

•Potassium supplementation may be necessary, as deficiencies can cause headaches.

•Drink lots of water if you are on the course and a headache appears. Dehydration can cause headaches.

•Ice cubes or a cold unopened can of soda on the base of the neck may reduce headaches.

•Alternative therapies such as Chiropractic and CranioSacral treatments may solve long-term headache trauma. Myofascial (muscle tissue) release therapy can be beneficial as well. Myofascial release has proven successful in relieving headaches, PMS symptoms, menstrual cramps, fibromyalgia and chronic fatigue syndrome.

•Folk remedy: Put an onion or horseradish poultice to the nape of the neck or the soles of the feet to relieve inflammation

•More supplements are discussed in Chapter 13.

Women may have an extra challenge on the golf course if they are pregnant, suffer from PMS, menstrual irregularities or menopausal symptoms. Many women have found wonderful solutions to reduce the unpleasant effects of the above, and their non-drug suggestions are incorporated into this chapter. Each woman's body is different; therefore, decisions on a selected course of action are individual. If you have an abnormal problem, it is essential that you seek proper medical care.

Help for PMS symptoms.

•Calcium/magnesium: may reduce symptoms over time. St. Luke's-Roosevelt Hospital Center in New York City discovered that administering 1200 mg. of calcium nearly halved PMS symptoms of the study subjects within three months.

•Consume carbohydrate-rich foods that may help reduce mood swings. These are considered to elevate levels of serotonin (a brain chemical that regulates mood), which normally diminish the week prior to a menstrual cycle.

•Expose yourself to sunlight. Please take care to protect your skin first with a proper UV-filtering sun-screen product. PMS mood swings that are elevated in the winter, may be caused by lack of full-spectrum light (light fixtures are available with bulbs that mimic sunlight). In a study by the University of California San Diego, women using bright white light for seven days prior to their periods had a lessening of symptoms.[13] It is thought that the light therapy may enhance serotonin production as well as regulating the body's circadian rhythms (the body's clock), both which can affect mood.

•Herbal supplements can reduce symptoms. Vitex (chaste tree berry) and maca are popular botanical herbs to treat PMS as it helps to restore estrogen/ progesterone balance. Clinical studies show that vitex reduces breast tenderness, bloating, fatigue, cravings for sweets, mood swings and depression. Dandelion can reduce water retention without depleting potassium stores (common in drug diuretics). Passionflower is a mild non-addictive tranquilizer, that may reduce headaches and cramping. *We recommend seeking the advice of a health practitioner before using these herbs if you are on the pill or are nursing.*

•Take supplements or eat foods rich in phenylalanine such as chocolate, turkey, pork, wheat germ and ricotta cheese. Phenylalanine is a neuropeptide

---

[13] For more information on light boxes & travel lights contact Apollo Light Systems (800) 545-9667 and SunBox (800) 548-3968

component and supports specific mood regulating neurotransmitters in the brain.

PMS Migraines.

•Migraines that sometimes are caused by excessive estrogen levels (which are often linked to birth control pills), may be helped by the following:

Suggested Preventive Migraine Formula:

•500 mg magnesium •99 mg potassium •1000-2000 mg bioflavonoids •100 mg vitamin B-complex • essential fatty acid supplement or flaxseed • 400 IU vitamin E •500 mg vitamin C.

Begin 1 week before your period and terminate 1 week after. If headache symptoms appear, double your dosage of bioflavonoids, potassium, magnesium and vitamin E.

•Increase intake of foods that have the amino acid tyramine, which affects the blood vessel tone and is found in foods such as pickled products, bananas, prunes, raisins, cheese, beer, wine.

•Herbal supplements such as feverfew, inhibit the release of blood vessel-dilating substances, thereby reducing headaches. Feverfew also helps reduce vomiting tendencies.[14]

•Reduce intake of sugars. Blood sugar imbalances can affect adrenaline levels and trigger migraines.

---

[14] Murphy, J.J., et al. Randomized double-blind placebo controlled trial of feverfew in migraine prevention. Lancet 1988 July 23:2(8604): 189-92

•Reduce intake of caffeine, an adrenal stimulant, as it may also provoke migraines.[15]

Pregnancy.

Most professional woman golfers do not excuse themselves from tournament play while pregnant. Nancy Lopez was a favorite expectant mother. And Tammie Green finished in the top 10 of 4 tournaments, plus she won the 1998 LPGA Corning Classic, and competed in the Solheim Cup, all while she was pregnant. Women surveyed who play while pregnant, agree that they felt an improvement in their games during this period. Anticipating the joy to come is a contributing factor, and let's not forget a potential physical advantage of having a lower center of gravity.

The exercise benefits of golf during pregnancy, particularly the walking, is beneficial for most. The only adjustment is getting used to squatting to tee the ball or pick it up. By the beginning of your third trimester, your swing will be greatly reduced as you get closer to your due date. During this time, it is important to avoid unnecessary twisting that can create trauma to muscles. You will be leaning over more to just see the ball, so don't strain your neck, either.

---

[15] Borok, G., et al. Migraine: treatment by personalized elimination program. Neurology Congress, March 1994

Additional nutritional suggestions:

•Drink as much purified water as you can bear. If you play in the heat, double your liquid intake and sit on the tee benches, if they have them. Electrolyte loss can affect your baby therefore drink mineral water often during the day.

•Bring along lots of fruit, particularly apples and other slow-release choices to keep you fueled. Snack whether you are hungry or not. Keeping ahead of the carbohydrate blood sugar swing will not only help your game, but make your baby happy, too.

•Choose an energy bar that has supportive nutrients for the brain such as flax, lecithin, gingko biloba herb, sunflower seeds.

•Choose afternoon tee times. Since some courses spray pesticides early in the morning, residue is more hazardous for golfers with early tee times. Pesticide ingestion from inhalation, skin contact or from putting your hands or golf tees in your mouth, is extremely hazardous to a fetus.

Menopausal symptoms.

Although there are a wide diversity of menopausal symptoms, each affecting women individually, we will only address the most annoying that we may experience during a game of golf, the hot flash.

•Avoid trigger foods such as tobacco, caffeine, spicy foods and sugar, as these elevate adrenaline levels that contribute to the hot flash.

•Maintain adequate levels of sodium, because deficiencies can also elevate adrenaline rushes.

•An over-estrogen condition can provoke hot flashes, as it keeps the body in a state of excitement similar to an adrenaline rush. This may occur when estrogen replacement therapy is not balanced by progesterone therapy. Estrogen levels may also be elevated because the body seems to recognize pesticide molecules as estrogen and reacts accordingly. If you eat sprayed or chemically treated food, be aware that this could elevate over-estrogen symptoms. To balance estrogen, apply a natural progesterone cream[16] to your skin each day for three weeks per month.

•Herbal remedies for hot flashes include combinations of dong quai, ginseng, hawthorne berry, wild yam root, chaste tree berry and licorice root. These are normally found in tinctures specifically formulated for menopausal symptoms.

•Vitamin E, along with vitamin C, can reduce hot flashes. Have your practitioner recommend proper dosages for your individual condition.

---

[16] Natural progesterone creams should include organically grown Mexican wild yam (Dioscorea) and Progesterone USP.

Chapter 12. Super Seniors.

Statistically, mature players are a visible force on links all over the world. Many chose to spend their retirement living in a golf community where back yards abut a favorite hole. Their numbers are well represented in tournament play, with some hitting their best games after the age of 50. Due to the inevitability of the body starting to show wear and tear, seniors tend to be the most concerned about prevention and healing.

Some of the pros have even taken to natural alternatives. For example: Bob Charles, the 63-year-old former British Open champion, attributes his longevity to supplements such as velvet antler and shark cartilage. Arnold Palmer and Jim Dent address arthritis with magnets or copper bracelets. We have already mentioned Gary Player, now in his 60's, and his total commitment to a sound diet. Six years ago, 72-year-old senior's trainer, Lee Bender, was walking around with a cane, suffering from gout and arthritis. Now he pumps iron for more than two hours several times a week in an organized exercise program. He attributes the improvement in large part to a change in his diet. Lee has cut back on red meat and eats vegetables, nuts, fruits and whole wheat breads, and in addition, takes supplements such as amino acids, alfalfa tablets and wheat grass. He claims to sleep better, have more energy, has lost his aches and pains, and continues to strive to reverse aging.

These seniors know that it's never too late to regain youthful energy and vitality. Age is not a determining factor in putting one's clubs away. Symptoms that include arthritic pain, pre-Parkinson tremors, back pain, osteoporosis and memory loss contribute to aging golfers abandoning the sport. Winning division tournaments into your 80's is not impossible, and if that is a goal, or if you just want to continue to play feeling well, then consider the non-drug suggestions that follow. As always, consult your health practitioner prior to any lifestyle or diet change.

Arthritis and joint stiffness.
•Drink the following liquids:

►Mineral water. Arthritis is thought to be caused by a toxic body trying to rid itself of waste particles. Minerals in water help this waste to move through the body, instead of ending up in the joints.

►Black cherry juice (best to use the concentrate diluted in water or juice) to reduce pain and swelling.

►Cabbage juice (you need a juicer for this) has been known to reduce the symptoms of arthritis.

•Consider taking supplements:

  ►Beneficial GLA (Gamma Linolenic Acid) from borage, Evening Primrose & black currant oils have shown to be effective in reducing inflammation and joint tenderness.

  ►Herbal remedies containing nettles, red clover, yucca/burdock, garlic, seaweed and nutritional yeast are great alternatives to a pain pill. Cayenne pepper capsules can bring blood to the joints and muscles to keep them warm and flexible, especially if you are living a sedentary lifestyle.

  ►Taking extra calcium and magnesium, and drinking goat's milk may improve the condition.

  ►MSM, (*Methyl Sulfonyl Methane*) is a naturally occurring, organic form of the element sulfur, which the body uses to create new healthy cells. As a supplement, it can be effective against arthritis.

  ►If you have bearing-down type of pain in the lower back, combined with a tired feeling, you may consider a homeopathic tissue salt: Calcium Fluoride which helps to preserve the power of elastic tissue to contract. Another remedy is Magnesium Phosphate, good for reducing steady, sharp neuralgic pains in the back, as it is an anti-spasmodic.

  ►Garlic, nutritional yeast and kelp can help reduce pain.

Osteoarthritis.

This is a condition that is characterized by the breakdown of the joint's cartilage, which causes the surface bone to rub against the opposing bone, resulting in pain and loss of movement. This disease normally affects the hands, knees hips, feet and back. Contributing factors are obesity, joint inflammation, chronic infections and years of repetitive use.

Supplement considerations:
•Herbal extract from the Rhododendron caucasicum plant has shown ability to inhibit collagen breakdown, (a contributing factor in joint trauma), thereby possibly acting to protect the body from osteoarthritis.
•Glucosamine sulfate rehydrates cartilage, giving it greater cushioning power, and may actually lead to the rebuilding of cartilage with long-term usage. It works best if used in conjunction with chondroitin sulfate. These substances can be found as supplements, or contained in Velvet antler. (Scientific literature from Russia, China and Korea reports the anti-inflammatory properties of antler velvet extracts, which could explain the traditional usage as a tonic for arthritis and similar inflammatory conditions.)

Tremors and shaking.

Contributing factors causing tremors as applies to the onset of Parkinson's, are hyperthyroidism, aluminum or heavy metal toxicity, pesticide residues, and various excitotoxins (example; MSG, aspartame).

Supplement considerations:
•Avoid foods high in chemical additives. Also implicated in symptomatic tremors are red wine, foods containing nitrate and nitrite preservatives, caffeine and drugs that cause blood vessels to dilate.
•Avoid excessive use of excitotoxins (aspartame, MSG, hydrolyzed vegetable protein, Hydrolyzed vegetable protein (HVP, which is used as a major ingredient for soups). Excitotoxins are additives that kill the nerve cells connected to neurons in our brain. This can create a domino effect, affecting nerves in other parts of the body. They can precipitate a fine tremor of the hands, and rigid, spastic-like movements of the body parts. (Parkinson's disease does not manifest until over 80-90% of the neurons in the involved nuclei have died. This takes years of assault from the excitotoxin ingestion to accomplish, therefore an occasional sugar-free snack or MSG-laden Chinese dinner will not create lasting effects.)
•Avoid anything containing aluminum, such as baking powder, and many calcium supplements, and some deodorant brands. This and heavy metal toxicity, which are suspect in brain disorders, have been implicated in pre-Parkinson tremors.

•Rhodiola Rosea herbal extract naturally stimulates the level of dopamine in the brain, which has been determined as a common deficiency in many pre-Parkinson patients. Studies have shown that this herb improves brain-cell activity, and helps the body to use oxygen more efficiently, increasing blood levels of specific brain chemicals. These brain chemicals relax us, and reduce the nerve-jangling effects caused by stress hormones.

•It is important to support the nerves and their neurotransmitters. This is best done with an essential fatty acid supplement, or by adding flax to your diet.

Osteoporosis.
This condition happens when the body fails to utilize calcium, which leeches out of the bone. It is marked by the appearance of small holes in the bones, and a generalized thinning of bony tissue.

Supplement considerations:
•Add supplemental Progesterone. Bone-forming cells come in two kinds: Osteoclasts (supported by estrogen) *dissolve old bone*, leaving empty spaces readying it for new bone growth. Osteoblasts (progesterone supported) move into these spaces to *build the new bone*. Too much estrogen (from estrogen replacement therapy or pesticides) without balancing with progesterone, stimulates the

osteoclasts, resulting in bone loss. It is prudent have a well-balanced hormone therapy program to reduce bone loss.

•Magnesium and calcium supplements. Magnesium is a carrier for the calcium on its trip to the bone. If too much calcium is ingested, it will actually cause a magnesium deficiency in the body. Low levels of magnesium can result in nervousness, fatigue, heart palpitations and depression. Boron is a naturally occurring trace mineral that should be part of any calcium/magnesium supplement. It decreases the urinary excretion of calcium and magnesium.

•Consider adding silica, which influences the uptake of calcium in the bones.

•Reduce use of sugar, sodas containing phosphoric acid, and the diuretic Lasix (consult your physician), as they may facilitate leeching calcium from the body.

•Using trace minerals, including copper, may facilitate calcium absorption. Too much vitamin A, E or potassium will upset calcium metabolism, and decrease its availability.

•Herbal treatments for bone support include wild oats, nettles, marshmallow root, yellow dock and horsetail (silica).

Memory and concentration.
An important part of any golfer's success depends on his or her ability to concentrate. Seniors seem to

forget things more often, and their focus may become less intense. Contrary to popular belief about these being indications of the aging process, they really are symptoms of nutrient deficiencies which compromise our thinking ability. Once these nutrients are restored, it's amazing how well our memory and concentration improves.

•Phosphatidyl Serine (PS) is a phospholipid that is particularly concentrated in the membranes of nerve cells and supports brain functions that tend to diminish with age. PS also may be related to the body's response to stress. As shown by studies, taking a PS supplement appears to produce fewer stress hormones in response to exercise-induced stress.

•Lecithin is produced by our livers, and is a major part of the brain. Lecithin is the major source of the neurotransmitter acetylcholine, which is the most important substance in nerve transmission. As we age, acetylcholine levels decline, leading to a reduction in both short and long-term memory. Deficiencies can hamper the proper operation of the brain. Extracted from egg yolks and soybeans, lecithin is easy to come by as a supplement.

•Herbal suggestions start with ginkgo biloba, which helps relax the muscles in our blood vessels, allowing more blood and oxygen to get to the brain. It also is effective for vertigo, dizziness and ringing in the ears. Newer research suggests that ginkgo also counteracts the sexual side effects of antidepressants such as Prozac and Zoloft. In addition to ginkgo, herbs such as anise, periwinkle, St. John's Wort, gotu kola, Siberian ginseng, wild oats, and rosemary leaves are helpful for memory retention.

•Dietary regimes should avoid allergenic foods such as sugar, wheat and dairy. Excessive use of aspartame sweetener should be avoided, as its long term use may change dopamine levels in the brain affecting memory, speech, vision and inducing headaches.

•Flax should be consumed daily, as it is high in essential fatty acids that are a key component to the operation of the brain.

•Mineral water or an electrolyte supplement can help remove heavy metal toxins from your brain. Heavy metals have been implicated in many illnesses, such as memory loss. A proper diagnosis of heavy metals in your body can best be determined through government approved laboratory hair analysis.

•Many emotional problems associated with memory failure can be treated with flower remedies (extractions from flowers, normally sold as tinctures). Flower remedies work quickly on the body chemistry that triggers emotions. The use of flower remedies can be effective in cases where the feelings of discouragement, failure, and frustration are present. They also seem to help motivation and concentration difficulties.

Heart.

Many cardiologists recommend golf as a method of exercise. Even if you do not have a known heart ailment, the following suggestions are beneficial as preventive "medicine". Doctors will prescribe foods to avoid, but it is up to each of us to follow their recommendations. Heart problems, in most cases, don't develop overnight. Many times it takes a scare, like a bad case of indigestion mimicking a heart attack, to make us pay attention to our diet. With all the media coverage on heart health, much information is available to help you protect yourself. We can suggest adding the following:

•Watching your diet and exercising have always been the rule and still are.

•Bioflavonoids are a beneficial supplement to guard against plaque build-up in arterial walls.

•Aged garlic extract has been found to lower LDL cholesterol, and it has been suggested that it may also slow the body's cholesterol synthesis.

• Herbs such as hawthorn berry and cayenne can protect the heart from various kinds of damage, including heart fibrillation.

•Essential fatty acids in the form of flax seed can reduce the build up of arterial plaque and protect against atherosclerosis.

•Mineral balance must be present to have any treatment be effective. Supplementing your diet with electrolytes can make the difference in the speed of any recovery.

•A specific antioxidant, tocotrienol, along with vitamin E, work directly against the action of the LDL (harmful) cholesterol. The tocotrienols are more effective at lowering LDL levels than vitamin E alone. Tocotrienols are found in grains such as barley, soybeans, rice, amaranth and others.

Chapter 13. Problem solvers.

Preventive medicine prepares your immune system to deal with stress, emotional conflict, competitive jitters, back pain, muscle strain and other maladies arising from a good game of golf. If you have a specific problem, you may want to consider using some of the natural treatments outlined in this chapter. This information is not meant to take the place of proper medical advice.

Anxiety.

•Avoid stimulants like caffeine, sugar and alcohol, as they will agitate your nerves.

•Herbal combinations of wild lettuce, valerian and cayenne supply nutrients to the nervous system to relax nerve fibers and reduce tension. Other useful herbs are scullcap, kava kava, and camu-camu.

•Use flower remedies for emotion. Whenever you tense up before a game, you can apply a specific flower remedy to your wrist or pop a few drops under your tongue. One containing aspen, mimulus, blackberry, cherry plum, red chestnut and rock rose should help to calm your emotions and relax you.

•Homeopathic Gelsemium can also have a calming effect.

Arthritis (pre-existing or ongoing condition).
•Use electrolyte supplement. For a more permanent treatment, take a mineral supplement or drink several glasses of mineral water every day. These will help to eliminate the debris which collects in your joints and causes inflammation.

•Plant enzyme supplements, taken when you eat cooked foods, will help digestion, thereby providing the immune system with nutrients to fight illness.

•Juices that help reduce pain and inflammation are black cherry and vegetable juice containing cucumber and cabbage (you need a juicer).

•Beneficial supplements are calcium balanced with magnesium, aged garlic extract, spirulina, algae, nutritional yeast, EFAs (supplement or flaxseed), and especially Borage oil (topically as well), and royal jelly (from bees). Vitamins E & C, niacinamide, zinc, velvet antler, glucosamine and MSM (methylsulfonylmethane: anti-inflammatory that strengthens connective tissue) are additional supplements that can reduce joint pain.

•Herbs such as devil's claw, yucca, comfrey, alfalfa, kelp, elder flower, linden flower, wintergreen, hops, scullcap, wild cherry bark and cayenne eliminate nutritional imbalances that contribute to arthritis and uric acid accumulation. Burdock, white willow bark, uña de gato, and ginkgo biloba reduce pain.

Back pain.

•Supplements that can assist in reducing back pain are vitamin B-complex with B_{12}, high doses of vitamin C, a calcium-magnesium supplement with boron for better assimilation, and co-enzyme Q10. To reduce swelling and inflammation, you can take Quercetin with Bromelain.

•Homeopathic Horse Chestnut sometimes eliminates the pain in 3-5 days, depending on the cause of the problem.

•Flower remedies can be used when emotional stress is suspected in causing the back pain.

•Herbal combinations of mistletoe, peony, cramp bark, lobelia, wild yam, gum myrrh, stinging nettle, skunk cabbage, scullcap and cayenne have been used to relieve muscle tension, aches and soreness.

Fatigue.

•Sugared foods or drinks should be avoided because of their unstable blood-sugar reaction.

•Electrolyte minerals in water are a superb alternative to high-sugar drinks.

•Reduce intake of foods that block iron absorption, such as sugared foods, beer, eggs and tea.

•Increase potassium intake to replace loss of potassium through dehydration. Use of diuretics or eating cooked foods will reduce your energy levels.

•Wheat and barley grass juice (in a supplement or energy bar) can be a great picker-upper before the game.

•While on the course, you may try flower remedies (topical or oral) specifically labeled for energy.

•Herbal combinations include gotu kola, panax ginseng, cassia, sarsaparilla, damiana, guarana, ginger, kola nut, ginseng and cayenne. Other individual herbs that can boost energy are Rhodiola rosea, gingko biloba, tribulus terrestris, mucuna pruriens, ashwaganda, maca, or velvet antler.

•Vitamin B_{12} is the "pep" vitamin. Vitamin C helps to maintain our energy supply and iron prevents weakness and fatigue.

•For a long-term sustenance program, add flax, nutritional yeast, chlorophyll, licorice, and calcium-magnesium to your diet.

Eye trouble: Good vision is critical to a golfer; therefore, it is important to give them dietary support.

•Electrolytes are essential for healthy eyes.

•Vegetables (raw or in juice) for preventive medicine diets include carrot, parsley, cabbage, kale, spinach, tomato.

•Supplements: EFAs (supplement or flaxseed), and zinc (for night vision), riboflavin (for cataracts), vitamin A (fish liver oil), lutein (balances vitamin A

intake), lecithin, bioflavonoids, amino acids, and supplemental oxygen.
•Herbs: cayenne (for circulation), bilberry (but not if you have Glaucoma), eyebright, and bayberry.

Female conditions.
PMS:
•Supplements: Calcium, magnesium, amino acid complex, bioflavonoids, EFAs (supplement or flaxseed), potassium, Vitamin E, C.
•Herb: feverfew for headache.
•Avoid stimulants such as sugar and caffeine to reduce headaches.

Pregnancy:
•Increase electrolyte water intake.
•Maintain complex carbohydrate (slow-release) diet to sustain energy level by eating during play, apples, grapes, unsweetened yogurt, slow-release energy bar.

Menopause (hot flashes):
•Herbal remedies for hot flashes include combinations of dong quai, ginseng, hawthorne berry, wild yam root, chaste tree berry (vitex) and licorice root.
•Vitamin E along with vitamin C can reduce hot flashes. Have your practitioner recommend proper dosages for your individual condition.

•Natural progesterone should be applied to balance estrogen levels, especially if you are on an ERT (estrogen replacement therapy) program.

Headache.
•Electrolyte water. Many headaches occur from being out in the hot sun, a result of dehydration. It is important to replace electrolytes lost by drinking lots of mineral water, before, during and after the game.
•Supplements for reducing incidences of headaches include bromelain, which acts like aspirin without risk of stomach upset. Niacin can help to keep the blood vessels and circulation open. Oxygen drops (found in health food stores) can help restore proper oxygen levels in the brain. Take potassium supplements if dehydration is suspected.
•Herbal treatments for headache include feverfew, valerian/wild lettuce, scullcap and gingko biloba.
•Trigger foods for headaches not associated with allergies or sinus: sugar, chemically-laced foods, additives such as aspartame and MSG and excessive alcohol.
•Small amounts of caffeine can sometimes relieve headache pain.
•An ice pack on the base of the neck may relieve pain.

•Acupressure points for headache include squeezing your thumb tightly against your pointer finger so a fleshy mound pops up on the back of the right hand between them. Now place the tip of the left thumb or knuckle, on top of that mound. Now relax the right hand and press the left thumb deeply into that area until it feels tender. The more it hurts, the more likely it is the cause of your headache.

•Aromatherapy treatments include applying lavender or peppermint oil on the temples.

•After the game, treatment for chronic headaches caused by muscle strain or back pain: physical therapy, chiropractic or CranioSacral treatment.

Memory and concentration.

•Electrolyte water. Again we stress the importance of supporting the brain with water containing electrolyte minerals.

•Supplements: Iron, (deficiencies can sometimes impair memory function), Vitamin B_{12} (builds the protein sheath surrounding nerve fibers. Deficiencies cause deterioration of the nerve tissue and may reduce memory function.), PS (phosphatidyl serine), lecithin, bee pollen, MSM, and flax.

•Herbs such as gotu kola, gingko biloba, aged garlic extract, and Rhodiola rosea.

•Avoid aluminum (baking powder, antacids, some calcium supplements, cooking utensil residue) and other heavy metals, as these have a detrimental effect on memory and cranial disease.

Mental acuity. Breaks in concentration can occur, even if one plays the game for years on the same course. Try the following:
•Electrolyte water. (creates the spark for brain cell transmissions)
•Supplements: EFAs (supplements or flaxseed), lecithin (supplement or as food ingredient), sea vegetable supplements (kelp, chlorella, spirulina), wheat and barley grass tablets or juice, thiamine, nutritional yeast (as long as you are not yeast-sensitive), phosphorus, bioflavonoids, Co-Q10, and B-complex, calcium-magnesium.
•Herbs such as gingko biloba, camu-camu, maca, ginseng and Rhodiola rosea.
•For on-the-spot mental boosts, try a flower remedy tailored for the emotions that counteract concentration lapses.

Muscle pain and sprains. It is prudent to first visit a physician specializing in treating these types of injuries. To further the healing process, you can support the body with additional nutrients.
•Electrolyte water. Since muscles depend on water for their operation, drinking plenty of water is

necessary to prevent the detrimental effects of any trauma.

•Supplements: potassium (lost from dehydration), vitamin C (increases the amount of glycogen stored in muscle tissue for energy, which can reduce the effects of muscle fatigue), vitamin E (helps prevent leg, calf and foot cramps), Calcium, (needed for muscle contraction, can quiet muscle cramps.), nutritional yeast (for those not yeast-sensitive), wheat and barley grass, glucosamine sulfate, MSM (methylsulfonylmethane: anti-inflammatory that strengthens connective tissue), magnesium, bioflavonoids, amino acids, bromelain enzymes, aloe (external), Co-Q10.

•Homeopathic pain relievers such as arnica, hypericum, rhus tox and ruta graveolens may be considered.

•Herbs: ginseng

•Flower remedies may give on-the-spot relief.

•Accupressure for relieving wrist pain, as well as certain pains in the elbow area, can be done while on the course. The spot is located by pressing deeply in the lower forearm, about two inches back from the crease of the inner wrist, in approximate line with the middle finger. Probe the area until you feel a dull, aching sensation.

Stress and irritability.

•Supplements: Thiamine (may steady nerves), vitamin A (counters the effects of adrenal stress), niacin (acts as a natural tranquilizer), magnesium (which is depleted during times of stress and needs to be replaced), vitamin C (A single outburst of stressful rage can burn up to 3 grams of vitamin C; therefore, if you are prone to getting mad during the game, carry your chewable Cs), potassium, zinc, lecithin, shark liver oil, calcium, pantothenic acid, B vitamins, aged garlic extract.

•Herbs: hops, passion flower, suma, astragalus, uña de gato, skullcap. ginseng, valerian, kava kava, St. John's wort, ashwagandha, maca, camu-camu, and Rhodiola rosea.

•Aromatherapy scents that are used for calming: lavender and ylang ylang oil.

•Flower remedies are extremely useful for any emotional outburst, and can have a calming effect almost instantaneously.

Upset stomach.
A bloated gassy stomach is no fun on the golf course. Antacids are very popular, and they may work temporarily. The body thinks antacids are food, and after the initial stomach acid is dispelled, the brain sends the signal to start the digestion process again. The stomach then produces more acid which signals you to take another

antacid, and another, etc. A better solution is to watch what you eat, so you don't get the stomach ache in the first place.

•Eat foods together that take the same time to digest, to avoid fermentation and gas. Basically, protein (meat) and starch (potato) don't go together, but vegetables go with everything. Fruit and dessert also, should be eaten individually as a separate snack or meal, without other foods.

•Antacid alternative: digestive enzymes available in pill or powder form. They help your stomach digest the food, and reduce gas and bloating.

SECTION 3. TRAVEL TIPS

Chapter 14. Travel health and golf.

Altitude.

You've just landed in Aspen Colorado for a golf vacation. After the drive from the airport and a hearty meal, you decide to take a nap. Twenty-four hours later you wake. What happened? If you are not used to the thin air of high elevation destinations, sleep becomes a very important part of your vacation. Normally, it takes about ten days to acclimate your body, but since your vacation ends before then, you may want to consider the suggestions in this chapter.

When oxygen levels are lower than those found at sea level, it stresses the ability of the cardiovascular system to deliver oxygen to the muscles when exercising. For two weeks prior to your trip, you may want to visit the gym, and indulge yourself in some high level aerobic workouts to prepare your lungs for breathing hard. The first symptom you may notice while huffing and puffing around a high altitude golf course, is increased respiratory rate. This normally begins within the first few hours of arriving at altitudes over 5000 feet.

If you are golfing at 8000 feet or above, you may be subject to symptoms such as headache, loss of appetite, fluid retention, an uneasy feeling, nausea and disturbed sleep. These symptoms usually go away in 72 hours after arrival, as your body adjusts to the thinner air. Factors that affect the severity of your symptoms are the specific altitude, level of exertion, and amount of hydration and diet. High fat and high protein diets increase the risk of susceptibility to altitude sickness.

To reduce the effects of these symptoms, you should limit your activity during the first several days. Relax and enjoy yourself for a day or two before tackling 18 holes of golf on an up and down course. Drink copious amounts of mineral and purified water to rehydrate yourself. If you develop a headache, you may take bromelaine or an herbal alternative such as feverfew. Exercise should be kept to a minimum during the period when the symptoms appear. An extra long sleep (12 hours recommended) may just be the easiest way to adjust to the altitude change.

For reducing the susceptibility to altitude symptoms, eat a high-carbohydrate diet. Carbohydrates require less oxygen for metabolism than fats and proteins. However, since a diet of only carbohydrates can unbalance the body, eat protein and fat on rest days. Avoid eating protein and fats at night, as these foods need extra oxygen for metabolism. When sleeping, the respiratory rate is already low, therefore you will be requiring more oxygen than is readily available, increasing the risk of altitude illness.

Heat.

Next on the list of golf destinations is a desert resort, and then on to the Bahamas. For both of these idyllic vacations, you may be dealing with heat that you are not accustomed to. Desert conditions may be hot and dry, while more tropical air masses are hot and humid. Obviously we all know that hot feels worse in humid conditions. But, hot is hot, and the suggestions for dealing with heat are the same.

We all have been schooled in the art of protecting ourselves from skin cancer and sun poisoning. SPF 30 and up sunblock lotions, plus wearing a hat, will safeguard your skin from the sun. The biggest risk to being outdoors in hot weather is heatstroke.

Children, elderly and obese people are extremely susceptible to heat-exhaustion, but golfers at any age who are moving around in the sun for 3 hours can equally be at risk. Contributors to heatexhaustion are cardiovascular disease, dehydration, drug usage such as amphetamines, excess clothing, prolonged exercise, sweat-gland dysfunction and alcohol use.

Initial symptoms of heat-exhaustion are dizziness, fatigue, muscle cramps, nausea, profuse sweating, thirst, weakness and lightheadedness. If you ignore these first signs, the illness could develop and you will experience cool, moist skin, headache, pale skin, nausea, vomiting, irrational behavior and eventually, unconsciousness.

If you do not get out of the sun and into a cooler area, you can develop heatstroke. Symptoms include dry, hot and red skin, fever above 102°F, dark urine, confusion, rapid, shallow breathing, rapid, weak pulse, seizures and unconsciousness. The most noticeable difference between heat-exhaustion and heatstroke is that in the latter, sweating ceases. Treatment for heatstroke includes getting victims into a cool place where they should lie down with their feet elevated twelve inches. Apply cool wet cloths to the skin, neck, groin and armpits. Give water with minerals or salt added (1/2 cup every 15 minutes). It is extremely important that you seek medical help immediately, as this condition can be fatal.

To protect yourself from heat-exhaustion, wear loose-fitting lightweight white clothes, rest frequently in the shade, drink plenty of water, and take your time getting around the course. Walkers may consider a cart during this extreme heat.

Air travel maladies.

The number one travel symptom, no matter where your final destination takes you, is jet lag. For those of you who travel east or west by airplane, you may experience various symptoms caused by your body clock's inability to compensate for shifting patterns of daylight.

In addition to a profound desire to sleep, or a bad case of insomnia, jet lag symptoms can include anxiety, body aches, coordination difficulty, disorientation, headache, impatience, inability to concentrate, indecisiveness, irrational behavior, memory loss and lack of sexual impetus. These are definitely unwanted on a vacation, or even a business trip in which you are fitting in a quick 18 holes between appointments. Some simple precautions can lessen the effects of jet lag.

Coffee drinkers will be happy when we say that caffeine can be medicinal. When taken in the morning, it can set the body's clock back, and when taken in the evening, sets it forward. Some travelers advocate eating only protein foods prior to your trip, other say to fast. It really is different for each person. We do know that dehydration aggravates jet lag, so carry lots of bottled water with you on the plane, and avoid all other liquids. One of the easiest recommended fixes for jet lag comes from the space program. A full spectrum (mimics the sun) light that you can take with you, when used in connection with a jet lag calculator[17], can reduce the effects of jet lag to one day, rather than the normal one to three weeks. You simply turn it on in the room for specific periods of time, outlined in the instructions, and soon your body clock is reset.

If you are prone to airsickness, you may want to carry ginger cookies, ginger spice or a ginger herbal extract. This herb settles your stomach. Sucking on a lemon or lime may also stave off the queasiness, as will dry soda crackers. Peppermint tea can also settle your stomach. A relatively new product at the airport newsstands, is an airsickness acupressure band that is worn on the wrist, and relieves nausea. If you are a fearful flyer, we have a proven remedy. A tincture made from the flowers of aspen, blackberry, cherry plum, garlic, mimulus, red chestnut and rock rose, seems to quell the emotions that trigger the fear. Available in specialty and health food stores, this flower remedy (see Resource Directory) is also beneficial for menopausal women who complain of panic attacks.

---

[17] For more information contact: Apollo Light Systems, Inc., Orem, UT (800) 545-9667

Golfing vacations are meant to be a pleasurable experience. If you plan ahead and prepare your body for climate changes or the stress of travel, you will arrive in fine shape to take on the challenges of new bunkers and water traps that lie in wait.

Epilogue

For golfers, each shot has the potential to provide tremendous satisfaction. That satisfaction will be much closer at hand if you nutritionally support that potential, both on and off the golf course. The foods we have outlined, as well as the herbs and supplements that fuel our bodies, will help us achieve maximum performance. By including foods that will deliver more consistent energy for stamina, mental acuity and muscle action, you will also benefit by controlling your temper and reducing the risk of ailments that can keep you at home in bed instead of on a sunny golf course.

Hopefully, you will find that nutritional comfort zone desirable and maintain this investment in your most important asset, yourself. Your golf game will definitely benefit and your overall health will extend your playing years.

Appendix A. Performance-enhancing supplements.

Please consult your health practitioner regarding proper dosages of supplements per your individual condition.

***Antioxidants*:**
Benefits: Stronger immune system, more resistance to colds, allergies, free-radical cellular damage from chemicals, pesticides, food additives, lowers serum cholesterol by interfering with its synthesis in the body, improves memory, enhances brain nutrition, prevents cancer.
Deficiencies: Lack of specific antioxidant foods in our diet and weakened immune system.
Sources: Vitamin E, C, beta-carotene, and garlic, which is used for colds, sore throats, topically to ward off wound infections, and as protection from virus, bacteria, parasites and fungus. Leave it to science to come up with odorless garlic supplements (aged garlic extract), which actually are more beneficial than raw garlic in many instances. Much research into the benefits of aged garlic extract (AGE) has been done, and we now know how truly beneficial this little clove is.

Another strong antioxidant is polyphenol, found in plants such as the Rhododendron caucasicum. Most of us have heard of proanthocyanidins, found in grape seed and pine bark. These types of antioxidants were thought to be responsible for the curing effects of grape seed. Proanthocyanidins are effective at helping cardiovascular conditions, but their large size prevents their absorption into the cell, reducing their antioxidant properties. A smaller, more absorbable form of antioxidant is a polyphenol, and when extracted from the grape seed or Rhododendron caucasicum plant, it can provide a superior antioxidant for the body.

Bioflavonoids. Referred to by some as vitamin P.
Benefits: An effective antioxidant, they also help alleviate the symptoms of asthma, assist in lowering cholesterol, protect connective tissue, and reduce bruising.
Deficiencies: Lack of bioflavonoid-rich foods.
Sources: Blueberries, cherries, turmeric, ginger, alfalfa, the white part under the skin of citrus fruits, certain herbs, bioflavonoid supplements.

Calcium
Benefits: In addition to building bones, calcium quiets muscle cramps, is essential for controlling anxiety and depression, and helps assure good sleep.
Deficiencies: Lack of calcium-rich foods, absorption interference from aluminum-based antacids, aspirin, cortisone, chemo-therapeutic agents, calcium channel-blockers and some antibiotics.
Sources: Dairy products, sardines, salmon, broccoli, dandelion greens, soy, collards, kale.
Caution: Calcium should always be taken with magnesium. There is a lot of hype on taking calcium supplementation to prevent osteoporosis, but rarely is magnesium mentioned. The latter is a carrier for the former; therefore, without magnesium, calcium won't make it to the bones. Silica also influences uptake of calcium. Taking too much calcium alone actually depletes the body of magnesium, and makes the calcium itself unabsorbable. Too much calcium can also disrupt the body's levels of zinc, iron and manganese. Suggested dosages: 1:1 ratio. If you take diuretics, you must add back the calcium, magnesium and potassium that is excreted.

Chondroitin Sulfate: (component of cartilage)
Benefits: Restores joints to original function, reduces joint pain, accelerates healing time for chronic arthritic conditions.
Sources: Supplements. Best results achieved when combined with Glucosamine Sulfate.

Chromium.
Benefits: Essential to the regulation of blood sugar, protects against cardiovascular disease, diabetes, high cholesterol, and helps to decrease body weight.
Deficiencies: Normally from eating white flour, milk and sugar, as those foods steal chromium from the body and excrete it unused.
Sources: Nutritional yeast, clams, honey, whole grains, liver, corn oil, grapes, raisins.
Notes: Nutritionally speaking, chromium is not well absorbed. As a result, a chelating agent or picolinate, needs to be combined with chromium, which allows it to bond with the other trace minerals.

Flower remedies. (Homeopathic extracts from specific flowers that treat emotions)
Benefits: Tinctures principally treat the personality state (mental and emotional) of a person. Many flowers will directly influence physical symptoms and disorders. Each flower has a distinct signature (smell, color, shape, location of growth), defining its particular therapeutic value. Flower combinations have the power to balance and change energy patterns in the human bio-electromagnetic energy field affecting mood, attitude and performance. Flower remedies are listed as to the malady you are trying to correct.
Sources: Supplements taken internally or applied topically.

Glucosamine Sulfate: (an amino acid formed in the body from glucose.)

Benefits: Necessary for cartilage rebuilding. Keeps joints elastic by restoring the gelatinous lubricating consistency of the fluids and tissues that surround the joints and vertebral areas. Helps with synthesis of collagen. Relieves pain and inflammation of osteoarthritis.[18] Alternative to nonsteroidal anti-inflammatory drugs.

Sources: Supplements

Herbs. Specific herbs are useful for increasing performance.

Gingko biloba is an important herb for strength, vitality, mental alertness, and to enhance vitality levels. It sends more oxygen to the brain for improved memory and brain function and is good for dizziness, vertigo and ringing in the ears.

Ginseng is the best known of the so-called aphrodisiac herbs, stimulates sugar removal from the system, improves mental states, assists memory, reduces depression, helps us deal with stress.

Kava kava and ginger work together to produce mild euphoria, and act as a relaxant.

Maca, a Peruvian herb, promotes mental clarity, increases energy and gives athletes stamina.

Camu-camu is effective against headaches and anxiety.

A combination of alfalfa, comfrey, gotu kola, peppermint, barley grass, spirulina, watercress, boneset and cayenne is used for regenerating bones, muscles, tissue and ligaments following injury or disease.

---

[18] Vaz, A.L., "Double-blind clinical evaluation of the relative efficacy of ibuprofen and glucosamine sulfate in the management of osteoarthrosis of the knee in out-patients" Curr Medical Research Opin 7: 104-14, 1981

Iron.
Benefits: Prevents weakness, fatigue, depression, dizziness, impaired memory, headaches, irritability and weak legs.
Deficiencies: Dietary. Aspirin and other anti-inflammatory drugs can cause iron depletion. Phosphates in sugar foods and beer can block iron absorption. Athletes working out more than six hours per week could deplete their iron stores and bring on anemia.
Sources: Molasses, cherries, prunes, leafy greens, poultry, liver, legumes, peas, eggs, fish, whole grains, herbs: alfalfa, bilberry, burdock, catnip, yellow dock root, watercress, sarsaparilla, nettles.
Caution: If anemia is not suspected, refrain from adding iron, as overdoses raise the risk of heart disease and colon cancer.

Lecithin. (A fat-like substance normally produced in the liver if the diet is adequate.)
Benefits: Dissolves the "bad" cholesterol in the blood, helps with memory loss, assists with absorption of fat-soluble vitamins because it's an emulsifier (makes two unlike substances able to merge), relieves angina and lowers atherosclerosis. Lecithin is necessary for the smooth flow of messages through the nervous system, thereby preventing disruption of muscle coordination.
Deficiencies: Dietary.
Sources: High-phosphatide soy or egg products. A thickening ingredient in many packaged foods. Supplements.

Magnesium.
Benefits: Assists in muscle contraction, lowers stress and PMS symptoms, guards against osteoporosis, muscle cramps,

calms nerves, reducing irritability, and is good for feminine menstrual cramps and nausea.

Deficiencies: Calcium/magnesium imbalance, dietary, sweat, urine.

Sources: Dark green vegetables, seafood, whole grains, dairy foods, nuts, legumes, poultry, hot, tangy spices, cocoa, supplementation.

Caution: See notes for calcium

MSM (methylsulfonylmethane), a natural source of sulfur. (Sulfur is critical in the formation of collagen and glucosamine, vital joint components.)

Benefits: Necessary for proper joint and muscle operation, treats arthritis, reduces the pain and inflammation of overworked muscles and joints. MSM has given positive results for osteoarthritis, and rheumatoid arthritis, acts as a muscle relaxant, eases stress, anxiety, depression and memory loss.

Deficiencies: Brittle hair and nails, arthritis, acne and depression are common indications of sulfur deficiency.

Sources: Milk, beans, garlic, onions, wheat germ, fresh fruit, eggs, meat and seafood, supplements (topical or oral).

Nutritional yeast. (Similar to Brewer's yeast but grown in a controlled environment and derived from plants, not hops. More nutritionally complete.) Yeast sensitive people may react to this supplement.

Benefits: It is a concentrated source of B vitamins and minerals (iron, potassium, calcium, chromium), and is a high quality protein with very little fat. Nutritional yeast contains quantities of thiamine, which can steady nerves. Excess sugar, alcohol and caffeine can deplete sufficient stores of thiamine and make golfers jittery during tense moments of play. Nutritional yeast also provides a good source of niacin

needed to control depression, irritability, and joint and muscle pain associated with athletic endeavors.
Deficiencies: dietary
Sources: Supplementation

Oil of Oregano.
Benefits: Reduces trauma from sprains, pulled muscles, leg cramps, muscle aches, carpal-tunnel syndrome and arthritis. Topically applied it can increase blood flow to the muscles and increase oxygen levels, which normalizes muscles.
Sources: Supplementation

Potassium. (an electrolyte that conducts electricity when dissolved in water.) Normal daily needs: 2400mg from all sources.
Benefits: Converts blood sugar into glycogen, which muscles use for energy, aids in sending oxygen to the brain.
Deficiencies: Dietary, lack of minerals in the water, sweat, stress, diuretics. If potassium is deficient it will affect the contraction process of the muscle, causing our muscles to tire more easily and become weak. Also contributes to poor reflexes and muscle damage.
Sources: Raw vegetables, fruits, citrus, lean meat, fish, beans and nuts, sports drinks.
Caution: Too much potassium in too short a period of time can cause cardiac arrest.

Rhodiola rosea.
Benefits: Contains active ingredients effective against heart disease, depression, cancer and stress, for treating memory, Parkinson's and as an aphrodisiac. It is used to enhance mental and physical performance, and to strengthen the immune system. Rhodiola rosea enhances performance by

decreasing the level of exertion of the regulatory system under physical stress. It also is an extremely effective fat-releaser providing "food" for our energy-producing molecules. Rhodiola also enhances a person's ability for memorization and prolonged concentration. In a proofreading test, those taking the extract decreased the number of mistakes by 88%.

Sources: Supplementation

Rhododendron caucasicum.

Benefits: Helps allergies, arthritis, various heart problems, and is a powerful antioxidant. It also is a fat-blocker, inhibiting the enzymes that digest fat, thereby preventing its absorption into the body. It is a proven anti-arthritic and gout, anti-inflammatory, anti-viral and anti-allergic herb.

Sources: Supplementation, Rhododendron tea.

Selenium.

Benefits: A free-radical scavenger, assisting in removing toxins from the body and repairing cellular damage, reducing muscle fatigue. If supplements are taken with vitamins A and E, it has been reported to help against breast tumors by promoting release of progesterone.

Deficiencies: In many areas of the country, this mineral is in short supply in the soil. Therefore, it may not be present in the food we grow. Deficiencies can cause cellular damage from prolonged exercise, resulting in muscle fatigue.

Sources: From foods that are grown in selenium-rich soil, supplementation.

Caution: Any supplementation should be done sparingly, as only trace amounts are needed to be effective. Not advisable to exceed 200mcg daily.

Sodium.
Benefits: Helps cells retain water and prevents dehydration. It also helps generate ATP (your body's energy maker).
Deficiencies: Exercising for long periods in hot weather, sweat.
Sources: Supplementation. Eating salt is not the answer, as the sodium in salt may not be bioavailable (absorbed) to the cells. Fluid-replacement drinks containing sodium.

Velvet Antler: (humanely harvested from elk antlers)
Benefits: Assists in prostate size reduction, helps arthritis, reduces osteoporosis, treats menstrual disorders, frigidity and infertility.
Sources: Supplements

Vitamin E:
Benefits: Excellent antioxidant, prevents cellular damage during exercise, prevents calf cramps caused by poor circulation in the lower leg, leg cramps and foot cramps. It can also help women with hot flashes and PMS.
Deficiencies: Dietary.
Sources: Wheat germ, sunflower seeds, almonds, pecans, peanuts, corn oil, peanut butter, lobster, salmon.

Zinc:
Benefits: Aids in post-exertion tissue repair through the conversion of food to fuel, helps with prostate problems, reduces inflammation, tones down body odor, boosts the immune system, prevents toxic effects of heavy metals like cadmium, improves fertility and sexual potency, reduces night blindness and reduces swelling and stiffness for arthritis sufferers.
Deficiencies: Over-exercise, lack of minerals in water or food. Studies correlate endurance exercise with periods of

compromised immunity, possibly because of zinc depletion. Constant aerobic training may accelerate zinc loss, and thereby put the athletes' immune system at risk. Zinc deficiencies can cause an imbalance in copper levels. When these are too high, they can contribute to hyperactivity and confused brain function, such as symptoms found in children with A.D.D.

Sources: Lean beef, liver, turkey (dark meat), pumpkin seeds, Swiss cheese, sunflower seeds, brazil nuts, oats, soybeans, peanuts, lentils.

Caution: Overdoses can lead to fever, nausea, vomiting, diarrhea, and cause iron and copper to leach from the body, contributing to anemia.

Appendix B. What *NOT* to feed your body.

What is not food, that comes in your food, but is really a chemical that can harm your body and reduce your competitive edge? We'll give you a little run-down on the things manufacturers do to your food to make it look prettier, taste better, last longer on the shelves and save them money. Do they really consider your health? Maybe so, maybe not. But why be the guinea pig? Here are a few of the culprits. You make your own decision.

Artificial color. Most people are aware of the toxic side effects of artificial colors and flavors from coal tar derivatives such as Red #40, a possible carcinogen, and Yellow #6, which causes sensitivity to viruses and has caused death to animals. Cochineal extract, or Carmine Dye, is a color additive used in food, drinks, cosmetics and to dye fibers red. It is made from ground-up female cochineal bugs from Central and South America. University of Michigan allergist, James Baldwin, M.D., confirmed cochineal extract triggered life-threatening anaphylactic shock in some people.

Aspartame. This very popular sugar substitute, known commonly as Nutrasweet, has very adverse effects on the human body. It contains Methyl Alcohol, a highly toxic poison that can cause recurrent headaches, mental aberrations, seizures, suicidal tendencies, behavioral disorders, birth defects, skin lesions and urinary bladder disturbances. The aspartame "hangover" may consist of malaise, nausea, headaches, dizziness, visual disturbances and convulsions. It has been implicated in Parkinson's disease and as a contributor to Alzheimer's. Aspartame has a detrimental affect on the neurotransmitter function, and therefore may be an underlying cause for interruption in concentration, focus and muscle control. For more information, read Dr. Russell Blaylock's book, *Excitotoxins: The Taste that Kills (see Recommended Reading list.)*

BHT/BHA. Used to stabilize fats in foods, these petroleum products have caused reduced growth rate in animal studies. Human reactions to BHA are skin blisters, infertility, liver and kidney damage, hemorrhaging of the eye, weakness, and discomfort in breathing. The International Agency for Research on cancer considers BHA to be possibly carcinogenic to humans, and the State of California has listed BHA as a carcinogen. Some studies show the same cancer-causing possibilities for BHT.

MSG. Most people are aware of the dangers of MSG and request it be withheld from restaurant foods. MSG, an excitotoxin, has been found to damage the retina of infant rats, and destroy nerve cells of the hypothalamus. Humans exhibit headaches, tightness in the chest and burning sensations in the extremities. Dr. John Olney of the Washington University School of Medicine in St. Louis, MO, notes that children are more susceptible than adults to the effects of MSG. Adults have well-developed blood-brain barriers that act as protectors from toxins. Children's brains are less fully developed. Therefore, with less protection, damage done to the brains of young children can be permanent.

Olestra. This is a new butter alternative, recently approved by the FDA. It is made from refined cottonseed oil and soybean oil, from which glycerin is removed and regular table sugar is added with the help of a catalyst. Since our digestive enzymes cannot break down the resultant sucrose polyester molecules, the olestra is reported to pass through the body undigested. This can cause gastrointestinal problems.

Found in breads, pastries, candy, and snack food, it is a potent allergen that can trigger anaphylactic reactions in people who have asthma or allergies. The Harvard School of Public Health states that "the long-term consumption of olestra snack foods might result in several thousand unnecessary deaths per year as well as causing diarrhea and other serious gastrointestinal problems." Even the label warns us against use: *Olestra may cause abdominal cramping and loose stools. Olestra inhibits the absorption of Vitamins A,D,E, and K and other nutrients.*

Pesticides. Found just about everywhere, including golf courses, pesticides are altering our genetic makeup, producing animal and bird mutations, and insuring the eventual demise of the planet. Most obvious is the assault to health, manifesting itself as cancer. Pesticides are implicated in the loss of sexual libido of both sexes. This is due to the fact that they mimic estrogen when absorbed into the body, and upset the normal hormonal balance. Fruits and vegetables that are most susceptible to contamination from pesticides (unless you choose organic varieties), in order of highest risk of contamination are: strawberries, bell, green and red peppers, spinach, cherries, peaches, cantaloupe (from Mexico), celery, apples, apricots, green beans, grapes, cucumbers.

Golfers should be particularly cautious not to put tees in their mouth after they have been placed in the ground, as has been the habitual stance for *Hal Sutton*. Also, when cleaning the ball with a glove, don't put the glove in your teeth to pull it off. It most likely has pesticide residue on it. If you are a smoker and have a habit of placing your cigarette in the grass while you swing, do not put it back in your mouth or you may ingest pesticides. We know of golfers who have been diagnosed with chemical allergy from pesticides, just from holding the club after setting it down on the green. Poisoning can come from inhaling or ingesting pesticides, but also from topical contact with the skin. If you really want to avoid the brunt of pesticides, take an afternoon tee time. Pesticide application to the course normally happens in the early hours around dawn. Early-morning golfers, therefore, are more susceptible to fresh pesticide ingestion, kicked up by their trek along the course.

Propylene glycol. Used as a de-icing fluid for airplanes, this chemical is added to food and skin products to maintain texture and moisture as well as inhibiting bacteria growth in the product. It also inhibits the growth of the friendly bacteria in your intestines and decreases the amount of moisture in the intestinal tract, leading to constipation and cancer.

THI (a browning agent). Cola drinks and processed brownish foods, get their color from an ammonia caramel compound called THI. The patent for THI is for its immune-suppressing qualities. Foods and drinks containing THI may look better, but by suppressing your immune system, can open the door for illness.

Appendix C. Foods containing specific nutrients.

Calcium: cheese, yogurt, sardines, milk, salmon, broccoli, dandelion greens, collards, kale.

Iron: beef, molasses, lima beans, sunflower seeds, fermented soy, prunes, turkey (dark meat), broccoli, spinach, almonds, peas, beet greens, nutritional yeast.

Magnesium: fermented soy, buckwheat, almonds, cashews, kidney beans, brazil nuts, pecans, whole wheat flour, peanuts, walnuts, banana, avocado, potato, oatmeal.

Niacin: chicken (white meat), beef kidney, salmon, brown rice, peanuts, nutritional yeast, sunflower seeds, milk.

Potassium: potato, avocado, raisins, sardines, flounder, orange juice, winter squash, banana, apricots, raw tomato, milk, salmon, sweet potato, apricots, peach.

Thiamine (vitamin B1): nutritional yeast, sunflower seeds, brown rice, salmon, peanuts, milk, chicken (white meat).

Vitamin A: beef liver, sweet potato, carrots, spinach, cantaloupe, kale, broccoli, winter squash, mustard greens, apricots.

Vitamin B_{12}: beef kidney, milk, chicken (white meat), salmon.

Vitamin B_6: salmon, peanuts, milk, chicken (white meat), brown rice, nutritional yeast.

Vitamin C: citrus fruits, Brussels sprouts, cantaloupe, green peas, strawberries, tomatoes, cauliflower.

Vitamin D: halibut, herring, cod liver oil, mackerel, salmon, tuna.

Vitamin E: wheat germ, sunflower seeds, nuts, cod liver oil, lobster, salmon.

Zinc: lean beef, turkey (dark meat), pumpkin seeds, chicken (dark meat), Swiss cheese, sunflower seeds, brazil nuts.

Appendix D. Fast and slow-release food listing.
(Random sampling)

Carbohydrates

High Glycemic	*Low Glycemic*
Fast release	**Slow release**
apricots	apple
bagel	beans
baked beans sweetened	brown rice
banana	buckwheat
beets	cherries
cake, cookies	chick peas
candy	citrus
carrots	corn
dates	fish
fruit in syrup	grapes
hamburger bun	green vegetables
ice cream	lentils
millet	meat
pineapple	milk
pizza	nuts
potato (baked, fried)	oatmeal
pretzels	oats
pumpkin	pasta
raisins	peanuts
rice cakes	pear
sugared cereals	peas
sweet corn	popcorn
tofu	rye
watermelon	soy milk
white bread	sweet potato
white rice	tomato
yogurt sweetened	yogurt (no sugar)

Appendix E. Foods necessary to treat the symptoms of a specific ailment:

Concentration
avocado
banana
beef (free-range preferred)
fermented soy
flounder
potatoes
prunes
raisins
sardines
spinach
sunflower seeds
trace minerals
water

Fatigue
avocado
bananas
chicken
citrus
fermented soy
lima beans
potatoes
prunes
raisins
salmon
sunflower seeds

Headaches
amino acid supplement
beef kidney
broccoli
brown rice
chicken
fermented soy
flax
lecithin
lima beans
milk
nutritional yeast
prunes
salmon
spinach
sunflower seeds
water

Muscle strength

avocado
chicken
citrus
cod liver oil
fermented soy
fish
flax
lima beans
milk
nutritional yeast
nuts
potatoes
prunes
raisins
salmon
sardines
sunflower seeds
water

Temper/impatience

carrots
chicken (white meat)
citrus
fermented soy
nutritional yeast
salmon
sunflower seeds

Appendix F. Quick-reference non-drug supplements that may help specific ailments (partial list).

Condition	Supplement
arthritis pain	aged garlic extract, green tea, jojoba extract, yucca extract, cayenne/ginger compress, flax seed, royal jelly, ginseng, CoQ_{10}, Rhododendron caucasicum herb, vitamin C, calcium and magnesium with boron, black cherry juice.
back & joint pain	MSM (found in milk, beans, garlic, onions, wheat germ, fresh fruit, eggs, meat and seafood), aloe vera, silica, comfrey herb, cayenne & ginger compress, L-Carnitine, bromelain, papain, vitamin C, calcium and magnesium with boron.
depression	amino acids, flower remedy, iron, nutritional yeast, magnesium, vitamin C, B_{12}, Herbs: Rhodiola rosea, St. John's.
fatigue	iron, flax, nutritional yeast, vitamin B complex, C, ginseng herb, spirulina.
heart	hawthorne herb, gingko biloba herb, evening primrose oil, potassium, aged garlic extract, cayenne herb, chlorophyll,

heart (cont'd)	CoQ10, vitamin E, trace minerals, magnesium.
irritability	flower remedy, iron, St. John's Wort herb, flax.
lower cholesterol	aged garlic extract, bioflavonoids, chromium, lecithin, nutritional yeast.
memory	lecithin, flax, amino acids.
menopause symptoms	vitamin E, natural progesterone, maca herb, ginseng, wild yam.
menstrual cramps	calcium, magnesium, maca herb, licorice herb, iron, vitamin E, flax.
muscle control	lecithin, potassium, selenium, trace minerals.
muscle cramps, spasms	calcium and magnesium, vitamin E, C, oil of oregano, iodine/potassium, horsetail herb, Rosehips, valerian herb.
muscle energy	potassium, trace minerals.
PMS	green tea, bioflavonoids, bayberry herb, ginger, burdock tea, wild yam, vitamin E, C, B-complex, flax, iron, magnesium.
stiff muscles	vitamin C, Rhodiola rosea, Siberian ginseng herb, potassium, tiger balm compress, cider vinegar and sea salt compress arnica (homeopathic).

stomach upset	digestive enzymes, ginger.
temper	flower remedy, kava kava herb.
tendonitis	bioflavonoids, alfalfa, ginger, cornsilk herb, rutin, vitamin C, niacinamide, trace minerals, zinc.
weight loss	chromium, Rhodiola rosea herb, Rhododendron caucasicum herb.
wrist spasm	ginseng herb, trace minerals, potassium, magnesium, valerian & wild lettuce herb combination.

RECOMMENDED READING:

Available in bookstores, or through the numbers listed.

The 8 Traits of Champion Golfers, Dr. Deborah Graham and Jon Stabler, (888) 280-4653, Published by Simon & Schuster

The Fitness for Golfers Handbook: Taking Your Golf Game to the Next Level, Don Tinder (888) 298-4122

Fit for Golf, Gary Player, Simon & Schuster. NY

Golf Begins at 50, Gary Player, Simon & Schuster, NY

The Secrets of Staying Young, Nina Anderson, Dr. Howard Peiper (888) 628-8731

Excitotoxins, The Taste That Kills, Russell Blaylock, M.D. Health Press, 1997

RESOURCE DIRECTORY

NATURAL PROGESTERONE FOR MEN & WOMEN. Useful in relieving the symptoms of menopause, lessens PMS, remedies osteoporosis, corrects mood swings. Natural progesterone (derived from wild Mexican yam) is a safe effective natural alternative to conventional HRT drug therapy. *ProgestaPlus*™ naturally restores critically important hormonal balance to help a woman regain her vitality, inner strength and youthful beauty. *ProgestaPlus*™' unique sealed pump dispenser delivers a fresh and correct dosage. AARISSE HEALTH CARE PRODUCTS, P.O. Box 210, Oakland, NJ 07436 (800) 675-9329 Email:jeff@aarisse.com www.aarise.com

CHLOROPHYLL PRODUCTS: DeSouza's Liquid Chlorophyll is a versatile product that can be taken as a dietary supplement, or used as a mouthwash and breath freshener. It contains no preservatives or flavorings, and comes in capsules or tablets. *TOOTH GEL,* is a breakthrough homeopathic dental care product that includes baking soda for whiter cleaner teeth, and potentized Cats Claw that is known for its positive effects on the gums, It is free from sodium lauryl sulfate and contains legendary alfalfa-derived sodium copper chlorophyllin, an excellent breath freshener. Also available is *DeSouza's ORAL RINSE and SPRAY,* an excellent cleansing agent, astringent and breath freshener with natural cinnamon flavor. Only the purest of water is used, with Ascorbic Acid added as a preservative, and it is alcohol free. DeSOUZA INTERNATIONAL, INC., PO Box 395, Beaumont, CA 92223 (800) 373-5171 www.desouzas.com

DAILY MAINTENANCE NUTRITIONAL SUPPLE-MENT. Two tables taken daily, of the DAILY MAINTENANCE FORMULA™ gives you a complete combination of vitamins and minerals necessary for balancing your body. A professionally formulated multiple vitamin-mineral supplement designed for long term nutritional maintenance and prevention. DAILY MAINTENANCE FORMULA™ may be used as a primary nutritional supplement. DAILY MAINTENANCE FORMULA™ provides maximum quantity of antioxidants, high levels of trace minerals, a full range of vitamins, excellent bioavailablity and a convenience of only having to take two tablets per day. HESED, Inc. P.O. Box 2002, Lenox, MA 01240 (800) 214-2344, or (413) 637-0067

FRESH FROM THE FARM. FLAX FOR YOUR IMMUNE SYSTEM. A whole food, *Dakota Flax Gold* is all natural edible fresh flax seed, high in lignins. Ready to grind, just like your best coffee, it is low in cadmium and is better tasting than packaged flax products. Seeds must be ground for full nutritional value. Dakota Flax Gold is available with grinder. Flax, also available in capsule form as *Flaxeon Jet,* is a convenient way of getting beneficial essential fatty acids. HEINTZMAN FARMS, RR2 Box 265, Onaka SD 57466 (800) 333-5813 (send S.A.S.E. for sample) Website: www.heintzmanfarms.com

VELVET ANTLER CAPSULES. Since *velvet antler* is said to build up the body's natural resources, it is becoming known as nature's perfect food. During antler growth, high levels of natural hormones are present in the blood, including IGF-I and II, which plays an important role in growth and development. *Velvet antler* is used to increase

physical endurance, sexual fitness, stimulation of the immune system, blood circulation, wound healing, energy, and for treatment of osteo and rheumatoid arthritis. MEADOW CREEK ELK FARMS, 7860 Woodland Lane, West Bend, WI. 53090 (888) 692-3113
website: www.elkantlers.com

DEAL WITH LIFE'S DEMANDS NATURALLY. Taken prior to a demanding workout, *Momentum*™ with Rhodiola Rosea helps muscles reach peak performance levels and delays fatigue. It also relieves daily stress, increases energy, vitality and alertness while improving mental performance and concentration, physical stamina and endurance.* The ultimate full-spectrum antioxidant *EnzoKaire*™ with *Enzogenol*™ (pine bark plus other OPCs) protects against free radical damage, reduces the effects of daily stress, increases energy and endurance, helps normalize inflammatory response and helps to maintain the structural integrity of joints. * *MSM Complex*™ support joint function and assists in cell permeability which allows pollutants from pollen, dust, mold and grasses to flow easily out of the body.* KAIRE NUTRACEUTICALS, INC., Longmont, CO (800) 870-0036 access code 167 or email: stephf@kaireint.com
www.kaireint.com

*These statements have not been evaluated by the Food and Drug Administration. This product is not intended to diagnose, treat, cure or prevent any disease.

FAST-RELEASE SPORTS BAR FOR QUICK START. Using fast-release energy carbohydrates and sweeteners, the *Stealth Bar* provides the best snack food for short-term energy. Combined with stamina-producing herbal ingredients it can deliver the power-boost you need to improve your game. KICX NUTRITION, INIC., 3210 20th Side Rd. RR 1, Campbellville ON L0P 1B0 Canada (905) 854-3572

FULL-LINE NATURAL SUPPLEMENTS . *Natural Factors* "takes their products right from nature to the marketplace". They control quality standards for every step of the manufacturing and distribution process, to fulfill their aim to "harvest, create and distribute the purest, most health-enhancing products in the world," according to Roland Gahler, President. Adding to their comprehensive line of vitamin, mineral, amino acid and enzyme supplements, *Natural Factors* also has a complete line of herbs, including those mentioned in this book; kava kava, Siberian ginseng, Panax ginseng, gingko biloba, feverfew, dong quai, cayenne, St. John's Wort and Valerian. They have supplements specifically designed for women, including Evening Primrose oil, a Woman's PMS Formula and Woman's Menopause Formula. For tackling specific joint and muscle problems, they supply chondroitin sulfate and glucosamine sulfate. To support proper brain health their lecithin, flax oil capsules and PS (phosphatidyl serine) are in an easy-to-take capsule form. *Natural Factors* has always had a reputation for quality, but maintaining that reputation requires a great deal of diligence, testing and investment in quality control. Even the finest organic ingredients must be thoroughly tested to ensure they meet *Natural Factor's* exacting standards. Their goal is to deliver products which marry the wisdom of ancient herbal physicians and the science of exciting, new clinical research to maximize the health choices of each and every one of their customers. Integrity means being able and willing to stand behind every product, a Natural Factor's commitment. Available in natural food stores. NATURAL FACTORS NUTRITIONAL PRODUCTS LTD. 3655 Bonneville Pl., Burnaby B.C., Canada V3N 4S9 (800) 663-8900 U.S. (800) 322-8704 located in Everett WA. www.naturalfactors.com

ALTERNATIVES TO DRUGS FOR HIGH ENERGY. *Medicine Wheel Herbal Drops* offer a variety of products. *HIGH ENERGY* includes herbs that aid acute exhaustion by supplying nutrients to the brain, circulatory system and muscles. *MEMORY BOOSTER* provides nutrients to the brain, increasing circulation and cranial nerve function. *Deva Flower® Remedies* reach the emotions surrounding symptoms. *FEARFULNESS*, effectively addresses fears of flying by directly bringing up and calming the emotional/mental issues that cause the fear. Also good for panic attacks. *STRESS/TENSION* eases headaches and clears mental strain and muscle tension. NATURAL LABS CORP., P.O. Box 5351, Lake Montezuma, AZ 86342 (800) 233-0810 Email: Natlabs@sedona.net   www.alternatehealth.net

IMPROVE FOCUS & CONCENTRATION. A convenient effervescent tablet that mixes with juice or water, can be your answer for sustained energy on the course. Pro-Endorphin™ contains DL-Phenylalanine (mood and concentration), B vitamins (stress reducer), DMAE (muscle coordination), Ginseng (stamina), Koal Nitada (blocks pain receptor sites), Inositol (brain food), Taurine (neurotransmitter modulator). Replaces electrolytes and sustains proper glucose metabolism. Excellent pain reducer for arthritis and muscle aches. Easy to carry in your pocket. NUTRACEUTICS, 3317 NW 10th Terrace, Ft. Lauderdale FL 33309 (800) 647-6377

SUPPLEMENTS FOR MENTAL ACUITY: *Trace-Lyte™* is a crystalloid (smallest form in nature) electrolyte formula that helps keep cells strong, balance pH, facilitate removal of toxins and provide the body's life force. If extra magnesium is required, *Cal-Lyte™* offers a 1:1 ratio of calcium/magnesium with boron to assist absorption. *Total-*

cium/magnesium with boron to assist absorption. *Total-Lyte™* is a 70% protein cracked cell yeast supplement that has been shown to increase mental efficiency, improve concentration, nourish the brain and combat fatigue. *Leci-Lyte™*, a unique blend of lecithin and crystalloid electrolytes, is one of nature's perfect brain foods. NATURE'S PATH, INC. PO Box 7862, Venice FL 34287-7862 (800) 326-5772, (941) 426-3375 Fax (941) 426-6871

RHODODENDRON CAUCASICUM and RHODIOLA ROSEA HERB. Caucasicum™ contains Rhododendron caucasicum, a lipase enzyme fat-blocker, and an excellent antioxidant, which contains grain kefir, containing 11 probiotics as well as a strong complex of minerals. Rhodiola rosea, found in *Z-1™* acts as a fat-releaser necessary for effective weight loss programs. QUEST IV HEALTH/ Donna Faucher, representative (888) 217-7233

ELECTROLYTE DRINK. *Golf-Lyte™* is an electrolyte drink that has no sugar or artificial sweeteners, dyes or preservatives. It contains true ocean-derived crystalloid electrolyte minerals (not sprinkled on trace minerals with electrolyte properties), and is in a base of pure oxygenated water, which helps to facilitate the body's ability to metabolize vitamins, minerals and other nutrients. The combination is unique and supplies a missing link. OCEAN-LYTE ENTERPRISES, P.O. Box 531, Jenison, MI 49429-0531 (888)-NUTRITION

BRAIN FOOD FOR HIGH PERFORMANCE. *Fortified Flax*, high in essential fatty acids, contains Organic Flax seed, Zinc, Vitamin B-6, C, E and is "yeast free". For a healthy snack, they also offer flax in a tasty *Omega Bar*, a convenient way to get energy. *Fortified Flax* can be sprinkled on cereal and sandwiches, or mixed with juice or water. OMEGA-LIFE, INC., P.O. Box 208, Brookfield, WI 53008-0208   (800) EAT-FLAX (328-3529)

TAKE YOUR NUTRITION ALONG FOR THE WORKOUT. *Pines Wheat Grass* and *Barley Grass* tablets are a convenient and natural way to get nutrients your body needs. In addition to naturally occurring vitamins, minerals, amino acids, protein, enzymes and chlorophyll, Pines International's cereal grasses contain fiber, which may aid in promoting regularity. After exercise, try *Mighty Greens*, a synergistic blend of superfoods, designed to provide high-quality nutrition, and containing herbs which may assist in fatigue reduction. PINES INTERNATIONAL, INC., P.O. Box 1107, Lawrence, KS 66044 U.S. 0(800) 697-4637 Canada: (888) 436-6697

ENZYMES FOR IMPROVING DIGESTION. *TYME ZYME™,* an all natural, <u>scientifically proven formula,</u> contains all the necessary enzymes (Protease, Amylase, Lipase, Cellulase and Lactase) for better digestion throughout the intestinal tract.   When taken with meals and/or supplements, *TYME ZYME™* increases nutrient absorption by up to 71%, and assures the body of receiving the benefits of vital nutrients and essential fatty acids. PROZYME PRODUCTS, LTD., (800) 522-5537 call Debra Casey for information.

Books from ATN/Safe Goods Publishing
Order line: (888) NATURE-1

For a complete catalog of Safe Goods books call (888) NATURE-1 or look us up on the internet: www.animaltails.com

---

Curing Allergies with Visual Imagery,
Dr. Wm. Mundy, $14.95

The Secrets of Staying Young,
Nina Anderson, Dr. Howard Peiper. $ 9.95

*Effective Stress and Natural Weight Management
using Rhodiola rosea and Rhododendron caucasicum,*
Dr. Zakir Ramazanov and
Dr. Maria del Mar Bernal Suarez $ 8.95

Plant Power,
Laurel Dewey $19.95

Self Care Anywhere, Gary Skole,
Vivienne Matalon, M.D., Michael Gazsi, N.D.,
Bruce Berkowsky, Ph.D., N.D. $19.95

Natural Solutions for Sexual Enhancement,
Nina Anderson, Dr. Howard Peiper $ 9.95

BIBLIOGRAPHY

-Aihara, Herman, *Acid and Alkaline*, George Oshawa Macrobiotic Foundation, 1986

-Anderson, Nina /Dr. Peiper, Howard, *The Secrets of Staying Young*, Safe Goods, 1999.

-Anderson, Dr. Richard, ND, NMD, *Cleanse & Purify Thyself*, R. Anderson, 1988

-Baldwin, James, M.D., *Cochineal extract*, Annals of Allergy, Asthma & Immunology, Nov., 1998

-Bolt, Ethan, *Muscles for Nothing, Strength for Free*, Men's Health, June 1999

-Burke, Edmund R., Ph.D., *What to do when exercise is through*. Nutrition Science News, May 1999

- Burke, Edmund R., Ph.D., *Nutrients Trim Injury Downtime*, Nutrition Science News, July 1997

-Burnett, Barry, M.D., *Diet Mania*, Nexus, July/August 1999

-Christianson, Alan, N.D., *Ten for the road. Essential nutrients for endurance athletes,* Nutrition Science News, May 1999

-Christianson, Alan, N.D., *Creating an Iron Man*, Health and Nutrition Breakthroughs, July 1999

-Coy, Chad, *Protein Powders: Whey to go*, Health Products Business p. 34, May 1999

-DuBelle, Lee, *Proper Food Combining W.O.R.K.S.* Lee DuBelle, 1987

-Gallon, Joanne, *Bar Stars*, Energy Times, July/August 1999

-Gittleman, Ann Louise, *Super Nutrition for Menopause*, Pocket Books, 1993

-Gleacher, Jimmy, *PS, Athletes Love You*, Natural Foods Merchandiser, July 1999

-Graham, Dr. Deborah, The 8 Traits of Champion Golfers, Simon & Schuster, Inc., NY

-Graves, Roger, *Alternate Shots,* Golf Magazine, Aug. 1999

-Heigh, Dr. Gregory, *Shopping to Avoid Genetically Engineered Foods*, Sun-Coast Eco Report, April/May, 1999

-Howell, Dr.Edward, *Enzyme Nutrition*, Avery Publishing, 1985

-Jensen, Dr. Bernard, Ph.D., *Chlorella, Jewell of the Far East*, Bernard Jensen, 1992

-Lee, Lita, *Prostate Problems*, Earthletter, Winter, 1993

-Liberman, Shari, PhD., CNS, *Nutrition Questions & Answers, New Life*, July/Aug. 1999

-Martlew, Gillian, N.D., *Electrolytes, The Spark of Life*, Nature's Publishing, 1994

-Meyerowitz, Steve, *Wheatgrass, Nature's Finest Medicine*, Sprout House, 1998

-Mindell, Dr. Earle, *Garlic, The Miracle Nutrient*, Keats Publishing, 1994

-Newman, Dr. L., *Make your Juicer your Drug Store*. Beneficial Books, 1970

-Null, Gary/ Null, Steven, *How to get rid of the Poisons in your Body*, Arco Publishing, 1997

-Platzman, Andres, R.D., *Friendly Colonization*, Food Product Design, Aug. 1998

-Player, Gary, *Fit for Golf*, Simon & Schuster, Inc., NY 1995

-Player, Gary, *Golf Begins at 50*, Simon & Schuster, Inc., NY 1988

-Ramazanov, Dr. Zakir and del mar Bernal Suares, Dr. Maria, *Effective Stress and Natural Weight management using Rhodiola rosea and Rhododendron caucasicum*. Safe Goods Publishing, 1999

-Rector-Page, Linda, N.D., Ph.D., *Healthy Healing*, Healthy Healing Publications, 1992

- Seibold, Ronald L., M.S. *Cereal Grass, What's In It For You!*. Wilderness Community Education Foundation, Inc., 1990

-Smith, Scott, *The Digest, Chew on this*, Golf Digest, Aug.99

-*Understanding Vitamins and Minerals, The Prevention Total Health System®*. The editors of Prevention Magazine, Rodale Press, 1984

-Winters, Catherine, *PMS Cures: help or hype?*, Fitness, July 1999

Index

151

152